I had brain what's your excuse?

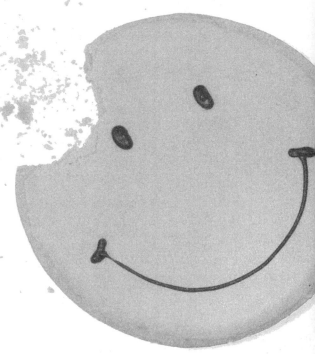

an illustrated memoir
by Suzy Becker

Workman Publishing • New York

For Pixie

Page 16. Drawings reprinted from *Neurologic Skills: Examination and Diagnosis*
by Thomas Glick, with permission of the author. *Page 65.* Excerpt from *Prepare
for Surgery, Heal Faster: A Guide of Mind-Body Techniques* by Peggy Huddleston.
Page 98. Lyrics from "Walking and Falling" by Laurie Anderson © 1982 Difficult Music,
reprinted with the permission of the author. *Page 126.* Photograph of Suzy Becker
© Liz Linder. Photograph of Herman Munster © The Kobal Collection. *Page 205.*
Photograph © Susan Wilson. *Pages 211, 259.* Cartoons by Suzy Becker first appeared
with *Gristmagazine.com.* *Page 226.* Lyrics from "The Ride" by Chris Smither © 1993
Homunculus Music administered by Bug Music, reprinted with the permission of the
author. *Page 242.* Excerpted from "What Does It Feel Like to be Brain Damaged?"
by Fredrick R. Linge, abstracted in *Canada's Mental Health* (September 1980).

Library of Congress Cataloging-in-Publication Data is available.

Workman books are available at special discounts when purchased in bulk
for premiums and sales promotions as well as for fund-raising or educational use.
Special editions or book excerpts can also be created to specification. For details,
contact the Special Sales Director at the address below.

Cover design by Paul Hanson
Interior design by Robin Ratcliff/Fyfe Design and Paul Hanson
ISBN-13: 978-0-7611-3979-9
ISBN-10: 0-7611-3979-6

Workman Publishing Company, Inc.
708 Broadway
New York, NY 10003-9555
www.workman.com

Printed in the United States of America

First printing: August 2005

10 9 8 7 6 5 4 3 2 1

ACKNOWLEDGMENTS

I do not want to give away the whole story before anyone gets to page one, but I will say, writing this book *was* my recovery. If it was ever possible to properly acknowledge all the help and encouragement I have received over the past four years, that possibility was ruined when I decided to change many people's names to protect their privacy.

My agent Edite Kroll, Peter Workman, and my editor Sally Kovalchick (who passed away the summer after my surgery) believed in this book from the beginning. I believed in them until I could believe in myself again.

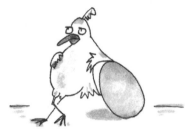

I have often been asked, "Which comes first, the words or the visuals?" And the answer is "yes." My editor, Suzie Bolotin, was patient, quick, smart, and funny throughout the whole chicken-and-egg process of making this manuscript into a book. Megan Nicolay is the world's best editorial assistant. Robin Ratcliff took a vision and expertly reined it in to design the book. I wish I could offer thanks both as enormous and complex. Thanks also to her assistant Anne Payne, and the rest at Workman: Paul Hanson, Paul Gamarello, Michael Fusco, David Schiller, Kim Hicks, Jim Eber, Gail Brussel, Patrick Borelli, Jarrod Dyer, Monica McCrady, Wayne Kirn, and Anne Cherry.

There were many tireless readers of this book whose enthusiasm and feedback sustained me through several revisions: Susan Anker, Robin Becker, Kathleen Cushman, Bill Strong, Susan Wilson, and Mako Yoshikawa. Alex Johnson's generosity with her time and her words moved me (and my book) further than she could have intended.

Karen Dukess's advice and friendship meant as much as they did freshman year when very little meant more. And Edite Kroll deserves a special award (or brain-cleansing and rejuvenating treatment) for the most reads, thorough edits, and pep talks.

I also want to thank Renny Harrigan, the Radcliffe Institute, formerly known as the Bunting Institute, and the Bunting class of 1999–2000. The fellowship made me write this book.

I will take another opportunity to thank my neurosurgeon Dr. Finn and his staff, especially Donna and Angela, the hospital records department, Dr. Hershorin and her staff, my speech therapist, Laura and Dr. Thompson, Ride FAR 6, and everyone I invited to the Thanksgiving brunch.

Bruce Kohl, Karen Simpson, Lois Becker, Alan Becker, Robin Becker, and Meredith Becker, thank you for the love and understanding that saw me through these worst of times. And thank you, Lorene, for the past two years with the promise of a happily ever after.

I have a terrible feeling I have forgotten someone, to whom I will owe an apology. There is no excuse.

Daily affirmation

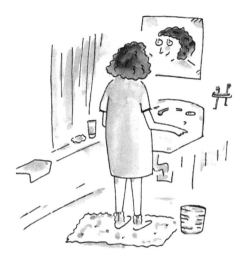

My life is interesting.
Others will find it interesting.
I would find it interesting if I weren't me.

Pre-Chapter One
PROCRASTINATION

TERRY GROSS (host of National Public Radio's *Fresh Air*): My guest is Suzy Becker, author of *I Had Brain Surgery, What's Your Excuse?* She is also the author of three other books, including *All I Need to Know I Learned from My Cat,* an international bestseller in the 1990s. Suzy, in addition to being a writer, you are a small-business owner, teacher—

ME: Was.

TG: —AIDS bike-a-thon organizer. Writing's not exactly a sideline, but your life isn't the quiet, contemplative writer's life some might imagine . . .

ME: I discovered writing at the end of my career as a cat whisperer—

TG: There's nothing about *that* in your bio.

I made it up—I'm making the whole thing up. It's a form of procrastination, I guess—making up interviews with myself on National Public Radio when I should be working on my book.

TG: I'm going to disappoint a lot of listeners when I admit I was *not* a fan of your cat book—I'm not a cat person or a big fan of gift books in general, or whatever they call that genre. Your new book is altogether different, not an *All I Need to Know I Learned from My CAT Scan* . . .

ME: It still makes a nice gift—*[wait, she should say that.]*

TG: It's nonfiction, very personal, a memoir of sorts. . . . People may think, brain surgery—who wants to read about that?! I wanted to tell you—I could relate to so much of what you wrote about and *I* haven't even had brain surgery! *[We laugh.]* You actually began working on this book while you were still recovering, is that correct?

ME: That draft ended up being more like notes than a book.

TG: I'm curious, at what point did you know—when the neurosurgeon told you you had a tumor and you were going to need brain surgery—devastating news for most of us—as a *writer,* was there some little part of you that said, "I'm going to get a book out of this"?

ME: Terry, I'm a writer, not an alien. *[I AM an alien. Writers don't waste valuable writing time making up interviews.]* I was devastated by the news. As a writer, I think I knew I'd write about it as a way to record the experience, maybe get some perspective, but . . .

Alien

TG: So, you were this perfectly healthy person: You were—I should say *are* athletic, you play volleyball, do these biking marathons, then in May of '99 you have a seizure. . . .

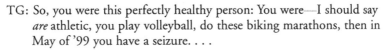

SNOWBALL in MIAMI

On April 29, I got this letter in my mailbox:

Radcliffe College

RADCLIFFE EDUCATIONAL PROGRAMS   RADCLIFFE INSTITUTES FOR ADVANCED STUDY

OFFICE OF THE PRESIDENT

April 27, 1999

Dear Ms. Becker,

I am very pleased to offer you an appointment as an Affiliate of the Mary Ingraham Bunting Institute at Radcliffe College for the 1999-00 year. Congratulations!

The chances of my receiving it were better than an appointment as Secretary of Defense—but only slightly. In fact, I never would have applied for a Bunting Fellowship if I had thought to fill out the forms *before* writing my project proposal.

I first read about the program in Mary Catherine Bateson's *Composing a Life* around the time I turned thirty. I loved Bateson's notion of life as a medium and the stories about her friends who had reinvented themselves as they got older. Bateson and one of the women got to know each other while they were Bunting Fellows.

I'VE ALWAYS WANTED TO BE MORE THAN ONE THING
WHEN I GREW UP...

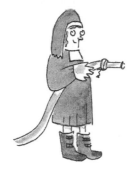

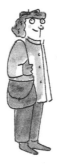

Age 5: NUN & FIREFIGHTER

Age 30: ENTREPRENEUR & AUTHOR/ARTIST

Each academic year, Radcliffe selects a community of three dozen scholars, artists, and scientists (primarily women) to work on individual projects at the Bunting Institute, a cluster of four pastel-colored Victorian houses on the campus. I associated the place with Bateson's book and mentally filed the fellowship under Inspiration, Reinvention, Friendship, and To Do Someday.

Five years later, I got up the nerve to request the application materials. I was in my second year teaching art at a charter school I'd helped to open. A rewarding, all-consuming job but, in my case, a noble diversion from a couple of my life's thornier projects.

A Bunting book project was a stone with two-bird potential. The one I proposed was *Fertile Mind,* a chronicle of my decision-making about whether or not to have a baby—in writing, cartoons, basal-body-temperature charts, graphs, newspaper clippings. SWF does battle with biological clock on a nonworking farm in the middle of Massachusetts. It was an obvious departure from my previous work, the embodiment (I thought) of founder Mary Ingraham Bunting's vision: "a shift into a different area of creative work at an early career stage."

I was pretty pleased with the proposal when I turned back to the forms. Two thirds of the way down the first page, I got to "Discipline Code (list only one)." *Do I put writer or artist?*

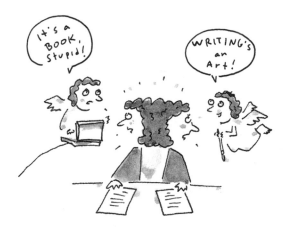

I finished the rest of the paperwork and came back to it. *They must make exceptions.* I called the Fellowships Office, and the receptionist put me through to the associate director.

"Do you consider yourself more one than the other?"

Well, yes, when I'm with writers, I consider myself more of an artist, and vice versa. . . . "I think I'm more of a humorist," I said.

"Humorist, hmmmm . . ." Very long pause. "The Bunting has never had one of those." I could hear the wheels of history creaking. "We had a comedian on staff once. . . . I'm not sure how to phrase this—we award the fellowships here on the basis of intellectual rigor. And I don't know whether we could call humor 'intellectually rigorous.'" *Too late to unpublish my pee and poop jokes.* "After all, our program is primarily for scholars."

I went back and forth, and on the last day, I decided to apply anyway. An out-and-out rejection couldn't be much worse than that phone call. *Discipline Code 6c: Creative Writing—Autobiography.* I drove my application into Cambridge and hand-delivered it. At this point I would have depicted my chances as a snowball in Hell, except Mrs. Geisman washed my mouth out with soap for drawing Hell in first grade.

MY CHANCES: SNOWBALL in MIAMI

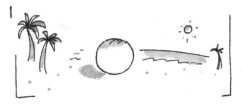

It is fair to say that the acceptance letter, a full seven months later, came as something of a shock to my system.

Mister and I celebrated for a half-minute when I walked in the door (about as long as he likes to stand on his hind legs), and then I called Karen.

"Guess what!"

"Suz, I'm late . . ." She was meeting some old college friends.

"I got it!"

"It?"

"I got the Bunting!"

"Ohmygod, I can't believe it, I mean—" She broke out laughing. "Suz, I am so proud of you!"

"Thank you. I mean, not for being proud of me—I think I might have quit if you hadn't read my application a hundred fifty times. . . ."

Karen and I had started dating a month before I talked to the associate director. More accurately, we'd gone out on one date and then spent as much time as we possibly could together. A variation on the classic "What does a lesbian bring on a second date? A U-Haul," since neither one of us was interested in moving.

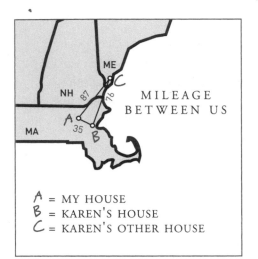

MILEAGE BETWEEN US

A = MY HOUSE
B = KAREN'S HOUSE
C = KAREN'S OTHER HOUSE

Karen is a graphic designer and historian. She was a seventh-grade history teacher who went back to get her Ph.D. at Tufts in the 1970s and ended up with an M.F.A. from the Museum School. When we fell in love, she was doing music graphics for record covers and publicity packages, giving lectures, and working on her third book about Boston's history. People used words like *lively, engaging,* and *fun* to describe her work—they describe her, too. And pretty. Karen would've been the teacher everybody had crushes on. (Grown-ups stood around after her lectures, like seventh graders after the bell, waiting to talk to her.)

When I was applying for the fellowship, it helped knowing that the Bunting had rejected Karen. For one thing, I could see *she* wasn't a loser. And she wasn't prone to false encouragement, even though we had just fallen in love. There were a couple of days when I was ready to throw the whole thing in the recycling bin and all she did was think out loud: *If I had a studio in Cambridge I could walk to her studio . . . we could have lunch together. . . . Some afternoons, we might just take off and go to the movies.* It made the dinkiest possibility worth pursuing.

Now she wanted to cancel her dinner plans. "We're celebrating!"

"We can't—you're already late, and your friends only get to see you once a year! Besides, I'm not letting you wait until next year to tell them about us. . . ." She groaned. It was her own fault for putting off telling them she'd broken up with her ex for more than a year. She could have had a hiatus, a year with no news, before introducing the new thirty-something girlfriend (me) into the midlife crisis picture. Karen was fifty-one.

"Maybe the fellowship will make me seem older or more serious or something." No response. "We'll celebrate this weekend."

"Promise?"

I promised without a twinge of disappointment. Celebration is a waste of early-stage euphoria. This is the time to do something so unpleasant you'd *never* consider doing it otherwise.

I picked cleaning the baseboards. I was up until 2 A.M., on my hands and knees, taking a toothbrush to the crevices in the kitchen and dining room. The next morning I was out in the garden before six. (Sleep is another waste.) I kept this schedule running for three days until I literally could no longer hold my head up. At a volleyball team dinner following an all-day tournament the night after Karen and I celebrated at the Charles Hotel, I rested my head on the

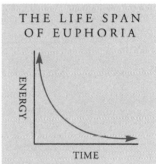

THE LIFE SPAN OF EUPHORIA

white tablecloth until the plates arrived. After espresso, I tried everything I could think of to stay awake on the drive back to Karen's: singing, counting backwards, chewing gum, driving with the windows open, biting my fingertips

I conked out immediately once I was lying next to Karen on the futon. Four hours later, I had a seizure.

> **grand mal seizure** characterized by the sudden onset of tonic contraction of the muscles, often associated with a cry or moan, and frequently associated with a fall to the ground. The tonic phase of the seizure gradually gives way to clonic convulsive movements followed by a variable period of unconsciousness and gradual recovery. (*Stedman's Medical Dictionary*, 26th edition)

The seizure I had in May 1999 wasn't my first; it was just the one that triggered the tests and everything else. I'd been having seizures for three and a half years—one every six months—which would have made this number seven or eight.

The first one was the scariest by far: September 1995. It was the month the charter school opened, which was the same month as Ride FAR (a biennial five-day, five-hundred-mile HIV/AIDS bike-a-thon I organize and ride in) and also the same month my third book, *My Dog's the World's Best Dog,* came out.

I was sleeping alone and woke up in the middle of the night—not wide awake, but alert enough to realize I was half-sitting and rigid. I couldn't straighten up or lie back down. I just half-sat there with no control over my body, thinking I was having a brain aneurysm. A friend of mine's wife died of one while he was out buying her a bottle of aspirin. After four years of walking around with this fear in the back of my mind, I was sure it had materialized.

I don't know what happened next. Whether I blacked out or fell back asleep, I woke up lying in a pool of urine. I turned on the light, put new sheets on the bed, and got back in the other side. I didn't call 911. I didn't call my boyfriend (who lived in the next town), or my sisters or my mother. I was *not* going to the hospital—no emergency brain surgery, *no thank you,* not for me. I'd take a chance on dying.

I lay there. My head ached too much to read. I tested myself by remembering the phone numbers of all the people I could have called. I did multiplication tables. I thought of one good thing from every year of my life going back to the age of two. The hours went by, and I kept watch, vigilant, never dozing. If whatever it was came back to finish me off, I was going to put up a fight.

After the sun came up, I showered, got dressed, and went to teach. I made it through the first day, thankful I didn't have a spaz attack in front of the kids. Then I got through the second day. And after a couple of weeks, I could almost convince myself the whole thing had been a bad dream.

TERRY GROSS: You showered and went to school the morning after what you described as a near-death experience: Did calling your doctor ever enter your thinking?

ME: Well, that's just it. I didn't have a doctor then. I'd never needed a doctor before—I mean, I knew I should have. A responsible adult *would* have called a doctor. And, that's partly why I didn't tell anybody in the beginning . . . plus I was afraid. . . .

Alien

I'm NOT an alien; a lot of people don't want to know what's wrong with them, especially if they think the best case involves brain surgery. I went to see a doctor a couple of months later. She said what I was describing wasn't a seizure after all, since I was awake at least part of the time. It was a stress episode. A normal reaction to book, school, bike-a-thon overload.

TG: Did she do any tests?

ME: No.

TG: What did she base her diagnosis on?

ME: My description, I guess. *[This is starting to feel like "Court TV," not "Fresh Air."]*

TG: Why didn't you get a second opinion?

ME: Because I think people get second opinions when they don't like the first one. I liked the doctor, and I liked her opinion—besides, it made sense. I always wondered where all my stress went. Turns out, I'm a repressed type-A personality. Nobody I knew—well, nobody I knew who knew—questioned the diagnosis. After I saw the doctor and everything was okay, I told my family and my boyfriend. It's not the kind of thing you go around blabbing about. I wanted to keep up my type-B appearance.

TG: Weren't you mad at the doctor once you found out?

ME: Everybody asks that. She'd moved to Chicago. I guess I could have stalked her . . . You want the real answer? *[Pause in case Terry answers.]* Sometimes I wish she'd never left and I could have gone on believing in her misdiagnosis for . . . ever. I would've rather had a seizure every six months. After the first few, I knew what to expect; the worst part was not knowing when.

After I stopped teaching in 1997, my life was a lot less stressful. I was writing and cartooning full-time (which felt like half-time compared with what I was used to). When the episodes didn't go away, I improvised on my diagnosis, updating the cause by substituting sleep deprivation, excess caffeine consumption, and euphoria for stress.

Date of Seizure: 1/16/99
Time: 2:40 A.M.
Place: Home
Duration: Less than 15 minutes
Description: Involuntary jaw movements and guttural noises; upper body convulsions; feels like heaving (without vomiting); fell out of bed; headache.
Cause: Memorial service 1/15/99. Karen's friend died of cervical cancer at age 35, following a misdiagnosis.

I had started to have doubts about my diagnosis earlier, but after the seizure that funeral night, they kept me awake. I hadn't been this afraid I was going to die since the first one. I turned on the light and woke up Mister. "It's okay, boy." He harrumphed and went back to sleep. Then I picked up the phone to call Karen. I didn't want to scare her; I just wanted to hear her voice. "It's me, sorry."

"What's up?" She almost sounded awake.

"I had one of those stress episodes." I had warned her about them when we started sleeping together, just in case. This was the first one since.

"Are you okay, Suz, is everything okay?" She was waking up. "What time is it?"

"It's almost three, Hen." Hen is short for Henny Penny. I'd meant Chicken Little when I came up with the nickname, but Hen stuck. "I'm okay. I think the funeral got to me."

"I wish I could've been there to hold you." She sounded warm and sleepy again. "I love you. Think you can go back to sleep?"

"Think so . . ." I turned out the light and fell asleep, wondering if I could.

The Bunting-acceptance episode in May of 1999 was the first anybody witnessed. My arms jerked so wildly, there was no way Karen could hold me. She was calling, "Suz, you okay? I'm with you—I'm right here." But her voice was barely audible over my own moaning; I hunkered down inside, waiting for it to end.

When I fell onto the floor, my arms were still. Karen knelt next to me and rubbed my back. I lay there; my tongue was too thick to talk. After a few minutes, I got up to vomit, and then it was over.

"Guess how long that lasted—until I hit the floor," I said.

"A half hour?"

"Less than ten minutes." I pointed at the VCR clock by the futon.

She didn't say anything. I went to lie down.

"Get dressed, we're going to the hospital."

No way. "I'm *not* going to the hospital."

"You don't have a choice." She stood up, and I lay down.

"Karen, it was a stress episode."

She didn't answer.

"I have an appointment with the new doctor in three weeks."

"We're not waiting three weeks." She held my chin and made me look her in the eye.

"I'll call in the morning."

She let go of my chin and came to bed.

I fell back to sleep with her legs tucked behind mine, a cure for my insomnia.

After breakfast the next morning, I called the new doctor's office. She could see me in three days, which gave me three days to brainstorm a list of *valid* medical concerns (something besides stress or appeasing Karen) that would justify butting in front of people who were *really* sick.

Valid Medical Concerns

spotting between periods

lower back pain

eczema (inner ear)

eyesight worsening

bunions

family history of osteoporosis and arthritis (prevention?)

family history of diabetes (causing stress episodes?)

~~stress episodes~~

OUT of the CLOSET

My new doctor's bio was hanging on the wall of her office:
M.D., Tufts '94, B.A. Biology, Brandeis '90, after taking five years off during college to work as an EMT. That made her (90 − 5 = class of '85) one
year younger than me. Her leisure activities included biking . . . I stopped
myself, I didn't want to be caught studying her bio.

In person, Dr. Hershorin was a good three inches taller than me and
wearing dress shoes, which made me immediately forget I was older. She
rolled a stool up next to where I sat at the end of the examining table on
top of the white paper runner with my paper robe crinkled under me.

I marked my place in my book and tossed it on top of the pile of
clothes on the chair.

"What are you reading?"

"Winter Birds."

"Any good?"

"Mm." I nodded. "A little grim." A very small inside joke with myself:
the author's last name was Grimsley.

She sat down. Her manner was calm. Focused, efficient, unhurried. A
good person to hear bad news from, although that hadn't become one of
my criteria yet.

"So, this wasn't your first seizure. . . ." she said.

"Technically"—I prefaced my three-and-a-half-year history with a correction—"they're not seizures . . ."

"I see. So, have you ever experienced any other shakiness or tremors in either side of your body?"

"Sometimes I have this tingling, I don't know if they're tremors—you can't see anything moving—on my right side, in my hands and my lips."

"How long?"

"Less than a minute."

She smiled. "I meant, 'since when?'"

"My teens. Early teens. But"—*I can explain*—"I was born six weeks premature. The pediatrician told my mother my autonomic nervous system wasn't quite fully developed. It's very sensitive."

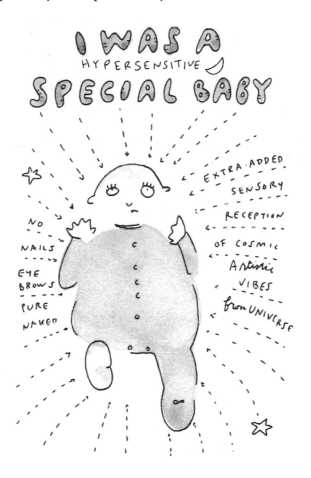

Dr. Hershorin did a basic neurological exam, a battery of a dozen or more rote-seeming tests that took less than ten minutes.

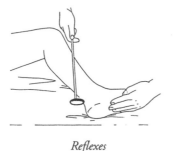 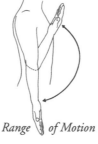 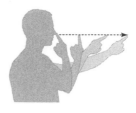

Reflexes   *Range \ of Motion*   *Hand-Eye Coordination*

I fished my list out of my back pocket while she finished writing on my chart. She looked up. "I'm going to order an EEG and a head CAT scan."

"But I passed all your tests!"

"The tingling you described is what's known as a 'focal seizure.' I want to rule out the possibility that something on the left side of your brain is causing all this." *Aren't those tests kind of expensive (I mean, I have insurance, but I'm not the kind of person who uses it) just to prove . . .* She interrupted my thinking. "We'll let the tests prove it's nothing." Her office scheduled them for May 19, six days before Karen and I were scheduled to take my mother to France.

My Seizure Druthers

1. Exhaustion

2. Random electrical storm

3. Epilepsy-mild

4. Epilepsy-regular

5. NOT Lupus or MS

In the two weeks between my appointment with Dr. Hershorin and the tests, I went from being a complete closet case to answering a passing "How are you?" with "I've been having seizures." You'd think it would be a conversation stopper, but it turns out everybody knows somebody who's had seizures and they're dying to talk about it. Somebody's ex-husband had the exact same kind as mine (the big ones) except his were during the day. He was diagnosed with a mild form of epilepsy and he never took the pills because he could feel the episodes coming on. Somebody's sister also had epilepsy and she never took her pills, either. Somebody's friend in high school used to have seizures, just from exhaustion, but they passed—the seizures, not the friend.

I didn't think much more about the tests themselves until a few days before I was supposed to have them. I had a mental picture of an EEG from an old *Brady Bunch* episode. For CAT scan, all I could come up with was an old cartoon I'd seen of a suspended cat—as in kitty—eyeballing the patient on the table. I was wishing there was a family doctor—a doctor in the family—I could call. Unfortunately, my family is in the furniture business.

I called Laura instead. She interned for me the summer before her senior year, then I hired her when she graduated, and we had been friends—unofficial family—ever since. Her father is a neurologist and professor at Harvard Medical School.

She had me call her dad at his office. When I asked Dr. Thompson what an EEG is like, he answered, "It depends what kind. Are you having a sleep-deprived EEG?"

I didn't know there were different kinds, and no one had said anything about not sleeping, but since sleep deprivation was one possible cause . . . I'd have to check into it. "And a CAT scan?" I asked.

"See if you can get out if it. You want to avoid radiating the brain."

THE INSURANCE HOOP

IF POSITIVE
Doctor needs to see more

CAT SCAN
*Required by insurer
(less $ than MRI)*

MRI

IF NEGATIVE
Doctor considers results inconclusive

I thanked him, forgetting exactly why I had called in the first place. I had no clearer picture of the tests, but I had a mission.

The receptionist in Dr. Hershorin's office took a look at my paperwork. "We have you down for a regular EEG." I asked her if she wouldn't mind double-checking and she put me on hold for a couple of minutes. "Dr. H. said if we need to, we can follow up with the sleep-deprived."

"I was just wondering"—*my mission was losing steam*—"if the CAT scan is, um, really necessary." It wasn't even a question. "I mean, could I skip"—*oh, she'll never go for "skip"*—"to the MRI?"

"You have the CAT scan and then we'll see about an MRI." No double-checking; I had wasted my option. I hung up. 0 for 2. *Somebody more assertive would have been able to score the sleep-deprived EEG, the MRI . . .*

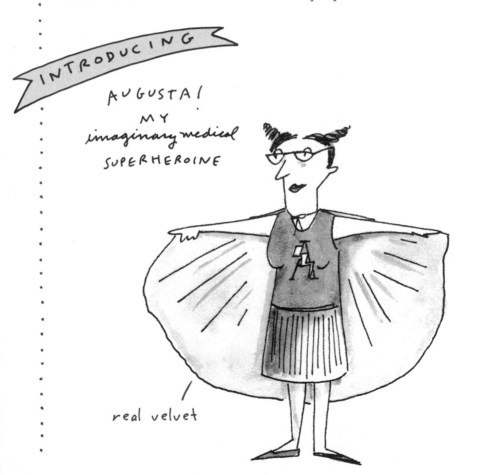

INTRODUCING

AUGUSTA!
MY
imaginary medical
SUPERHEROINE

real velvet

Karen took the morning off to come to my tests. I had said it was not really necessary—I wasn't going to be getting any results or anything—but, now that we were in the hospital, I was glad she was there.

The clerk at registration typed in my information, never taking her eyes off the screen.

"Emergency contact?"

"Karen Simpson."

"Relationship to you?"

I paused.

Possible answers:

(a) friend

(b) ~~g~~girlfriend UNCLEAR *as in* "I went to the mall with my girlfriends."

(c) partner *seems premature for 9 months*

(d) significant other *too Cambridge*

(e) lover *Yes, we _do_ it.*

The clerk rested her palms on the desk and finally looked up.

"Partner." The clerk looked at Karen. Karen looked pleased. It was the last question.

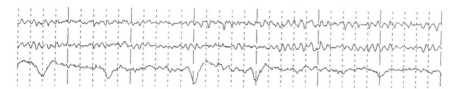

In the meantime, a man from the EEG department had arrived to take me down for my test. Karen's on-the-walk interview revealed he'd given up a position teaching art at the high school for this "more lucrative, more monotonous" position at the city hospital. I would have guessed FM DJ from the gravelly voice and the long gray ponytail.

Coincidentally, his department looked a lot like a radio station or a recording studio. EEG Man worked in a darkened control room filled with blinking machines (no windows, except the one looking out on the testing area) and an intercom system. He sat me down on the bed. Then he separated my hair, put a dab of petroleum jelly on my head, and mounted each electrode. It felt pleasant, like I was getting my hair done. But, then again, I'm A.H.D.D.

Attention to Hair Deficit Disorder (A.H.D.D.)

<u>History:</u> Patient's two sisters had long, luxurious straight hair that invited/required brushing. Patient's short wavy hair invited sisters' brushing into Wolfman hairdo when parents were out.

<u>Behavioral Observations:</u> While patient exhibits low tolerance for styling own hair (she has not owned a comb or brush since 1983), patient continues to exhibit a high (at times inappropriate) tolerance for others' attention to her hair and head.

<u>Impressions and Recommendations:</u> Patient suffers from low hair-self-esteem. She is inclined to experience any attention to head (e.g., EEG) as pleasurable. Patient may benefit from a haircut. She should also be encouraged to keep some hair equipment in the house for own and guests' use.

The EEG Man asked me about my seizures while he was doing my hair. He had a new diagnosis: sleep behavior disorder. "You see it more with kids, boys, mostly, who get up and go to the bathroom in their bureau drawers." *Bureau-wetting . . . something else to worry about.*

After he affixed the last electrode, he had me lie back and guided my head down to the pillow. Then he went into his control room.

The EEG was as relaxing as a test can be—all I had to do was lie there. About two thirds of the way through, he announced over the intercom, "These strobe lights sometimes set off a seizure; try to stay relaxed." The lights flashed for a while and nothing happened. Then he had me breathe in and out as fast as I could and I felt the tingling on my right side.

When we were all done, I asked him if I'd had a "focal seizure" during the breathing part. He said the only irregularities he had detected were some sleep-type brain waves—consistent with a sleep behavioral disorder. At least it didn't sound fatal.

The electrodes took a lot less time coming off. When he was done, EEG Man offered me his comb (I passed) and a souvenir printout page from my test (I accepted)—a gift from a former art teacher to a former art teacher. Then he walked me back to the waiting area.

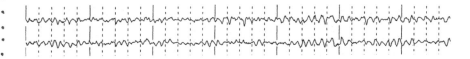

Karen had written down the directions to radiology. All hospitals are mazes, I've since concluded; the most poorly designed non-English-speaking airports are easier to get around in. We made a bathroom stop on the way so I could check my hair. It was like we'd stepped back in time. The floor was covered with tiny white hexagonal tiles. The fixtures were from the 1940s, big fat enamel toilet bowls and sinks complete with rust stains—the kind I would've liked in another setting, a restaurant or an old train station, but I found them unsettling in a hospital. "I'm sure they put all their money into machines," Karen suggested.

When we got to radiology, I gave my name and they handed me a clipboard with a three-page questionnaire. I filled in the answers while Karen read her magazine. After I returned the clipboard, I scanned the waiting room over the top of my book—*sick or just waiting? sick or just waiting?*—until my name was called. GAME OVER!!!

The nurse began by apologizing. She was new. Then a second apology: "I'm sorry, Suzanne, but we're going to have to go over all these questions—

what she says:

Suzanne.

what I hear:

SUZANNE ROSE BECKER YOU COME DOWN HERE THIS INSTANT! Your father is going to hear about this!

standard procedure here at the hospital. They don't want to miss anything."

"Suzy," I said. She apologized a third time and made a note of it.

I sat on a table, actually more of a gurney, with my back to the CAT scan, a machine with an opening the size of a laundromat dryer. She read off each question, the whole question, no shorthand, on the three-page questionnaire. She was remarkably enthusiastic about this part of her job. "Are you allergic to any medications?"

"Yes, sulfa," I said, "and," I added, even though it wasn't a medication—her enthusiasm must have inspired me to share more—"shellfish."

"Shellfish! Well, I'm glad you told me, Suzy, because sometimes, not very often, the doctor will want to do a dye-injected CAT scan and it's not un-usual for people who are allergic to shellfish to be allergic to this dye. It's iodine-based. But, like I said, the doctor doesn't use the dye much and, of course, we have another dye we can use."

Maybe you should put "shellfish allergy" on the questionnaire. "Why would the doctor do a dye injection?"

PARTS OF
THE BODY

"It can give him a better reading . . . it depends on what he sees *up there*." She smiled.

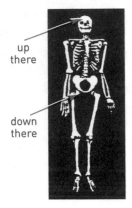

up
there

down
there

New Nurse asked me to lie down. She stressed the importance of keeping my head completely still while she wedged foam rubber around my neck. Then she handed me a set of earplugs, no explanation. As soon as I had them in, she strapped my arms down and hurried out of the room; I figured we must've gotten behind going over the questions. I lay completely still with my ears plugged and my arms strapped down.

Ask her what to expect. NOW!!!

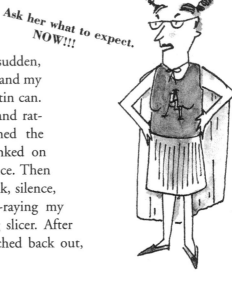

All of a sudden, the table lurched backwards and my head was inside a big shiny tin can. Seconds later, the banging and rat-tling began, which explained the earplugs. The machine clanked on for five minutes. Then silence. Then lurch. I was farther in. Clank, silence, lurch; the machine was X-raying my head like a hard-boiled-egg slicer. After five or six slices, I was lurched back out, and New Nurse reappeared.

"All done?" I asked.

"The doctor," she said as cheerily as ever, "would like to do a dye-in-jected scan." She loosened the arm straps and swabbed the veins in my left arm with rubbing alcohol, while she explained the benefit of a dye-injected

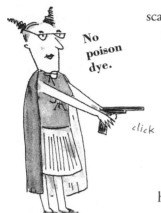

No poison dye.

click

scan, as if I'd never heard of it. Then she picked up the needle and uncapped it.

"Isn't there a test, something you do to see if I'm allergic to the dye?"

She had to take the cap out of her mouth. "Goodness, that's right! I'm glad you reminded me. Shellfish! I don't know the answer to that." She scurried out of the room. Seconds later she scurried back in. "We don't have a test. There is no test for that. I shouldn't have told you. The allergy is very, very rare."

"What about the other dye?"

Back out of the room. Back in, this time with an old nurse, her supervisor. Old Nurse spoke, "We don't have that dye here. If you want it, I will have to go somewhere else to find it and you'll have to go back to the waiting room. It could take several hours. I can't tie up my machine."

"Okay. I mean, I think I'll wait. I'd like to try the other dye."

"One in one hundred thousand people are allergic to this dye." *Correction: one* is, *not* are, *allergic.* Old Nurse got closer. "One in one hundred thousand is nothing. And the other dye, *if* I can find it, is also more expensive. Your insurance may not cover it."

"How much?"

"Eighty-five dollars."

Eighty-five dollars?! Eighty-five dollars is nothing! The way she was peering down at me made me flinch. "What *kind* of allergic reaction is it?"

"Anaphylactic." Her tone had turned soothing, "We'd know in the first sixty seconds, and we're right next door to the emergency room here."

"Okay, go ahead. I'll try it." New Nurse swabbed again. I felt the prick—*fifty-nine one thousand, fifty-eight . . . fifty-seven.* She missed the vein. Take two. She missed again. *Let's get the Russian roulette over with!* I turned to Old Nurse. "You do it. You need to find the vein this time."

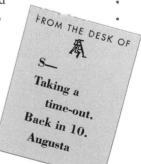

FROM THE DESK OF

S—

Taking a time-out. Back in 10.

Augusta

New Nurse looked relieved. Old Nurse hit the vein and the dye went in. I could feel the warmth spreading down through me.

"The dye can make you feel like you're wetting your pants," Old Nurse said after the sixty seconds had passed.

"Am I?"

"So far, no one has." She slid the needle out. I checked my pants, then she strapped my arms back in and the two of them left the room.

The second round didn't take as long. New Nurse sprang back in the room—"All done! Wasn't so bad." She started unstrapping—the table jolted back again. She shoved my head down before it hit the machine.

"What's happening?"

"I don't know!" She sounded panicky. This time she ran out of the room. She'd collected herself by the time she returned. "The doctor just wants to take a few more pictures!"

Sirens were wailing in my head. *He sees something.* "Does he see something? Do you know what he sees?" She left the room without answering.

It had finally gotten through my skull: *Something is wrong.* New Nurse would not offer up any information. "Your doctor will have the results on Monday."

I practically ran to the waiting room. Karen wasn't where I had left her. The back of her Laurie Anderson hair was bobbing down the hall. I wanted to shriek, "Come back!" but I stood there frozen, waiting.

"They saw something!" I told her everything the second she came back. She very calmly reassured me it was nothing. Just their incompetence. "Of course these bozos aren't going to get it right the first time or the second . . ."

And I believed her.

CALL ME FERDINAND

Two days later (the Friday before the Monday my results were due), I was back in Dr. Hershorin's office for the appointment I'd originally scheduled regarding Valid Medical Concern #1, before I had the seizure or the tests.

She opened my folder. "I'm going to write up an order for a pelvic ultrasound, just to give us both peace of mind." She didn't have to explain this time: she liked to order tests to prove it is nothing, not because she suspected it is something. She handed me a copy of the order and started to close the folder. "Looks like we have your CAT scan results!" She wheeled over closer so we could both read:

Valid Medical Concerns
~~spotting between periods~~
lower back pain
eczema (inner ear)
eyesight worsening

```
CLINICAL HISTORY: SEIZURES

WITHIN THE LEFT PARIETAL LOBE, THERE IS A FOCAL AREA OF ENHANCEMENT
MEASURING 1.1 CM X 7 MM IN SIZE. THIS AREA OF ENHANCEMENT COULD BE
SECONDARY TO REACTIVE HYPEREMIA FROM A SEIZURE FOCUS. A MASS CANNOT
BE EXCLUDED.  THERE ARE NO DRAINING VEINS OR SUGGESTIONS THAT THIS
IS VASCULAR IN NATURE. THE REMAINDER OF THE INTRACRANIAL STRUCTURES
ARE UNREMARKABLE.

IMPRESSION:
1. 1.1 X 7 MM ENHANCING REGION INVOLVING THE LEFT PARIETAL LOBE AS
   DESCRIBED ABOVE.
```

I never got past, "A mass cannot be excluded." (I didn't take in the part about how the rest of my brain structures were "unremarkable.") "What does this mean?" I thought I was dying. *I'm going to be sick. I better stand up.*

"Wait right here; I'm going to call the neurologist." *See? She thought it was nothing. She was not prepared for this development.* I sat back down and concentrated on not being sick. I could hear her voice through the door, so I knew what she was about to say, "The neurologist is gone for the day *and* he's on vacation next week, but I'm going to track him down. I'll have an answer for you before I leave here tonight." I stood up to go.

"Will someone be at home with you?" I nodded. "Is there someone you'd like to call?" I shook my head no. *I'd like to get out of the office without having a breakdown.* I walked to my car, shoved Mister over, and got in.

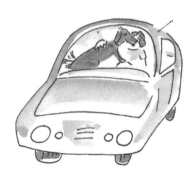

SYMPATHY OR SALT LICK?

I stopped at a phone a few blocks away. Karen was in Maine. Her machine answered. I left a neutral message, and then I tried my sister Meredith. She picked up, and at the sound of her voice, I started to cry, which made her cry.

It was a minute before either one of us said anything. "Mer, they think I have a mass in my head."

"Oh. Oh. Oh. All right. A mass. Okay, what does that mean exactly?"

"I don't know. She didn't know. I'm just scared; I didn't know I was going to find out—I have to drive myself home. . . ."

"Stay there; I'll come get you." She was in Springfield, two hours away.

"That's ridiculous." It made me stop crying.

"I'll come over tonight."

"It's okay, Bruce is coming."

"Does he still have my clothes?" When my friend Bruce and I helped her move in the fall, he offered to take a couple of bags to the Salvation Army. They were in the trunk of his car.

"Did you want your prom dress back?"

She laughed.

"I'm okay to drive now." I promised to call her later.

By the time I got home, both Karen and Dr. Hershorin had called. Dr. H. said I needed an MRI right away.

"June seventh's the earliest," I told her. "I get back from France—"

"When do you leave?"

"Tuesday."

"You around this weekend?" *You're making this sound like an emergency.*

"I have volleyball championships tomorrow."

She'd schedule the MRI for Sunday. And the neurologist wanted me to start taking antiseizure medication immediately.

"Should I cancel my trip?"

"Don't do anything *yet*." She caught herself. "Suzy, don't get too worried about all of this. Let's wait until we have all the information. Try to have a good weekend. Good luck with the championships. I hope your team wins."

Karen wanted to drive back from Ogunquit. I convinced her to stay; she doesn't see well at night, and it didn't make sense when I'd be playing volleyball all the next day. She'd come home Saturday afternoon, as planned, and we would go to my MRI on Sunday.

I called in the prescription. And I made one more call to Bruce; he said he'd leave work right away. Then I put the phone back in its cradle. I had forty-five minutes of alone time with my news.

What does *this mean? It doesn't mean I'm dying. Whatever it is, this mass on the left side of my brain, it is not killing me. It's had at least three and a half years, maybe twenty-three and a half to finish me off. It's free-loading, along for the ride. Every six months, we go through a little readjustment, but in general, it's live and let live.*

The MASS in my HEAD

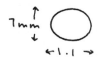

Its dimensions weren't very impressive. In fruit, vegetable, or sports ball (the usual lay diagnostic) terms, I was looking at an underdeveloped grape. I decided to call it Ferdinand, after the pacifist bull. Ferd for short.

THE PARIETAL LOBE. I checked the small dictionary. The medium dictionary. The big dictionary. My college human physiology textbook. My *Scientific American* brain book.

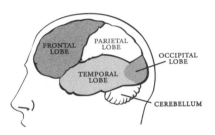

Location, location, location. *But, what does the parietal lobe* do? I couldn't find anything in any of the books. No personality traits, behaviors, bodily functions. Not your major league lobe—part of the 90 percent we don't use on the side that handles accounting, neatness . . . They could probably remove the whole thing and I'd be no worse for wear. But no one had said anything about removing anything. *Yet.*

I put the books away. That was enough alone time, however much time that was. I picked up the phone, then put it back down. Seizures were one thing, easily forgotten; but a mass in my head . . . every time I'd run into somebody:

It's SUZY with the MASS in her HEAD—I must ask her...

How ARE you, really?

There goes poor SuZy with that mass in her head.

Isn't that SuZy? Her head doesn't *look* any different...

I had come dangerously close to creating a loop—every call I almost made would have required a call back with MRI results, for starters—and I did not want to be in the loop-maintenance business.

I checked the kitchen clock; it was after 6:30. Bruce was due to arrive any minute. Then maybe we would go get the prescription. Not the most exciting Friday night, but it would make the annals.

BRUCE & SUZY's EXCELLENT ADVENTURES

motion odyssey movie at Jordan's Furniture

wed. nites at the Elks Club

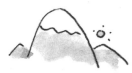

Death marches and bike rides

Dairy Queen season openings & closings

Backyard luau (his 30th)

PLUS the night I found out I had the MASS in my head...

Bruce was an hour late, which gave me a lot of time to think about the prescription. We could still go get it, but I wasn't going to start taking it, not right away. I didn't want to be logy for the championships. And I didn't want to be drowsy on top of jet-lagged in France. Besides, I am not a pill person—I wasn't discriminating against the medication—I don't take vitamins, either. Yesterday I was fine; today I need to be medicated immediately. *I don't think so.* If I wasn't careful, this thing could take over my life.

Bruce arrived in his work clothes. We hugged, and I got dark tearstains on the shoulder of his French blue shirt. "Sorry, I'm late, Suz. I called Bill—then the traffic was horrible. He said to say hi, and if you want to talk about any of this . . ."

Bill, Bruce's boyfriend of several months, lived in California. I hadn't met him, never talked to him; still, it *was* a nice offer, and coming from someone who'd had a brain tumor—that was one of the first things Bruce had told me about him (the coincidence now struck me). But all I had was a *mass.* And I wasn't interested in talking about it. "Do you know anything about the parietal lobe?" I asked.

Einstein's inferior parietal lobe was 15 percent wider than normal, with additional claims that the cell density was higher, permitting enhanced usage or more interconnections.

"I think Bill's was in his pituitary. We could look it up on the Internet." I shook my head: too much information. "Isn't—there was something on NPR—I think Einstein's parietal lobes were bigger than normal. . . . They didn't say what they do."

"Oh, yeah," I said in this singsong mock-cocky tone we sometimes use with each other, "extra mass in my parietal lobe, I'm a genius. . . ."

Bruce drove to the CVS. By then, neither one of us could say the word *antiseizure* without faking a seizure. When we stopped for gas, a guy held the door for Bruce. "You look like you're in a hurry."

"My friend just found out she has a mass in her head—we're not sure how long we've got . . ." he said, and ran back to the car. We laughed hysterically at this. We laughed hysterically at a lot of things that don't seem so funny now.

The two of us split up in the CVS parking lot. Bruce went to the supermarket to get the makings for dinner, and I went into the pharmacy.

"Five bucks if you sign for the prescription like this," Bruce said, faking another seizure.

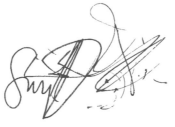

"Ten." Five was so cheap. He made thirty the last time we were at dinner—a hand clasp (ten dollars) and a kiss (twenty) for the birthday woman at the next table.

The ten was lost the second I stepped inside the CVS. It was like a chemical reaction to the fluorescent lights. My stomach knotted up while I stood waiting in line, and when my turn came, I signed, didn't ask any questions, paid, pivoted, and exited down the nearest aisle, just like the people in front of me.

Bruce didn't bring up the bet. We had dinner and played Yahtzee. I would've sworn it wasn't my lucky day, but dice don't lie. I got two Yahtzees. And the next day, we won the volleyball championships.

In the gym, I flipped back and forth between the two channels in my head. Without the volleyball channel, it would have been all mass, all the time. This way, at least half the day, my mind was on other things.

BECKER TELEVISION

	8:00	8:30	9:00	9:30	10:00	10:30	11:00	11:30	12:00	12:30
COURT	Volleyball		Volleyball		Volleyball		Volleyball		Volleyball	
OFF COURT	Mass in My Head		Mass in My Head			Mass in My Head			Mass in My Head	

Karen hugged me so hard when I presented her with my championship jacket, I thought for a second she regretted missing the finals. Then I remembered: She hadn't seen me since the mass.

I took a long bath; we got mediocre Italian food and went to bed. I slept surprisingly well, exhausted, content, relieved she was next to me again.

The next morning, I got out of bed early to give myself extra time to think about my outfit. (Usual time = 0.) The incentive: If you don't wear metal, you get to keep your own clothes on.

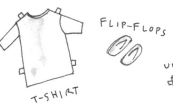 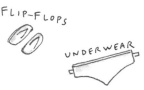 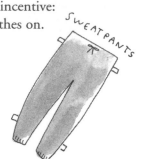

The MRI suite was in a "mobile unit" in the parking lot behind the hospital. The place was in Sunday mode, deserted. They let Karen come back with me.

The nurse immobilized my head in a futuristic catcher's mask. And this time, I had a choice: radio or earplugs. Radio was the obvious choice.

Inside the machine, a tiny rectangular mirror above my head showed the rest of the room *upside down.* Karen was sitting in a ɹIAHƆ, holding my foot, keeping up both sides of a conversation. I closed my eyes and flashed for a second on the rust-stained toilet bowls. *They put all their money into machines; they put all their money into* sǝNIHƆVW.

The radio came on and drowned Karen out. Radio in a tin can, all of a sudden, seemed so obviously a bad choice. Top 40 (mixed with static) blared six inches from my ears; I couldn't even feel Karen's hand on my foot anymore. I opened my eyes, and she was gone from the little mirror. She had to be checking out the control room.

The machine started ticking—its resting pulse—then a buzzer went off, an old recess buzzer, the edge taken off by snippets of Top 40. I closed my eyes and tried to think of peaceful things: *earplugs; having a normal Sunday; going for a bike ride; knowing nothing was wrong; going to France knowing nothing was wrong—but if something was wrong, going to France knowing nothing; putting it out of my mind and dealing with it when I got back.* Karen was back there, trying to find out what I did *not* want to know. The next time the buzzer stopped and the ticking started, I looked for the nurse in the mirror. I'd forgotten her name. "Excuse me, is it almost over?"

"It's taking a bit longer than normal."

That set the sirens off in my head. "Are you seeing something?"

"Your friend is talking to the technician."

"Tell her to stop talking." I had to yell to be heard. "Please!" Karen slid back into her seat.

When it was over, I beelined for the front office without looking sideways at my brain on the monitors that filled the control room. Karen stopped to say good-bye to the technician. On the trailer landing, she announced, "I saw it! She showed it to me. It's filled with fluid." *Fluid? Is it an aneurysm? No, a cyst. A fatty cyst. The kind they leave in.* "The technology is so fascinating."

Fascinating? FASCINATING?! I know there are people who would request the video of their own colonoscopies, but—*I'll tell you what I'd find fascinating:* NOTHING. *A big fat fluke.* "What did she think it was?" I asked. She didn't know.

We were almost at the car. "Will we be able to go on our trip?" Karen hadn't asked. I was quivering, just this side of crying. "I wanted to go away *not* knowing. And, now, we don't *know* anything; we just know it's bad."

"Suz, you should've told me."

"I didn't know." I was crying.

"I was only doing what I would have wanted you to do." Now she was crying. "How could you not have known? The CAT scan—"

"You said it was the bozos." I caught my breath. "A mistake . . ."

THE REGENERATION OF HOPE

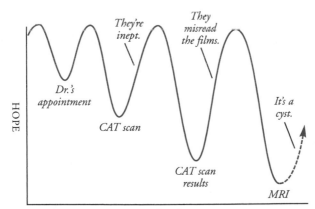

The GOOD
BAD-NEWS DOCTOR

The next afternoon, I ran from the car to the house, trying to keep my new traveler's checks out of the pouring rain. There was one message on the machine. "Suzy, this is Laura Hershorin. Please call the office *immediately.* I have your MRI results."

The MRI confirmed a mass in my head. She had called Dr. Cook, the best neurosurgeon in the area (he had operated on Michael J. Fox), and he could squeeze me in at the end of the day—which meant I needed to leave *now.* I called Karen; she'd meet me at his office. Next, I needed to find myself a ride; even if it *was* safe for me to drive I-had-no-idea-where *with* the mass and the rain, there wasn't enough time to park, get the MRI films from the hospital, *and* be at his office by five.

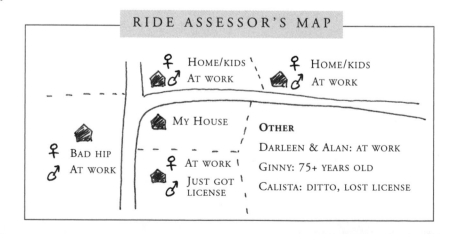

RIDE ASSESSOR'S MAP

♀ HOME/KIDS
♂ AT WORK

♀ HOME/KIDS
♂ AT WORK

🏠 MY HOUSE

OTHER

DARLEEN & ALAN: AT WORK

♀ BAD HIP
♂ AT WORK

♀ AT WORK
♂ JUST GOT LICENSE

GINNY: 75+ YEARS OLD

CALISTA: DITTO, LOST LICENSE

I called a stranger, a friend of a friend who came to mind only because she had left a message the week before (not like her, she said), suggesting a dog walk or something so we could get to know each other. She (no small children) runs a business out of her home in Bolton. Someone else answered. "Cathy can't come to the phone right now. May I take a message?"

Shit. "It's urgent." It was worth a try.

"This is Cathy Freed." It worked!

Keep it light. "It's kind of a bad day for a walk, but I was wondering if you would be interested in a drive—I'm supposed to be at a neurosurgeon's in Lowell at five. I, um, just found out I have a mass in my head."

No questions, she'd be right over. I wanted to run out and wait for her, in the rain, in my bare feet. *Think sensibly.* Shoes. *Not your sandals, cover your toes.* Raincoat. Directions. Paper. Pen. Put Mister in the mudroom. *Where is she?* I felt like crying. *Think sensibly.* Turn on the outside lights. Inside lights. *You're acting like you're not coming home.*

Well, am I? Do you know? What if he needs to operate immediately? It's already dark out, and I am trying to think—feed the cat—*sensibly.* When Cathy arrived, I ran out and flopped in the car.

A dark car ride is an underrated way of getting to know someone. Better than a dog walk, less eye contact than a cup of coffee. In between driving instructions, I told Cathy everything that had happened so far, up to the fluid-filled mass in my head.

"I know someone who had an aneurysm." She paused. "Do you want to hear?" *I don't know—does it have a bad ending?* "She's fine." The gist of it was her friend had survived the brain surgery. At first she had trouble reading, but now she's back at work. The conversation turned to talk of our town; polite at first—we both regretted the lack of diversity.

"But we *do* have people of color," I protested. "Bob Welch—"

"Planning Board?"

"Yep. He's practically purple." It felt good to laugh. She double-parked by the hospital entrance, and I literally ran through the rain to radiology and back. The directions to Dr. Cook's were now soaking wet. We were lost within minutes. After we stopped twice to ask for directions, Cathy finally pulled into a U-Haul center, marched through the puddles, and came back with a map.

We were only fifteen minutes late. Cathy got us each a cup of water, and we had just sat down next to a couple discussing a disability claim, when Karen walked in and walked right by us. I caught up to her at the desk and tapped her on the shoulder. "Oh, my god, I thought I was so late. The traffic—oh, I'm so glad!" She hugged me, and I introduced Cathy. Cathy, who now knew me way better than she'd bargained for, hugged Karen hello, good-bye, and was gone.

Around 5:30, Dr. Cook came down the hall to greet us. "Well, you've got the bad news"—he sounded very upbeat—"but as far as bad news goes, it's pretty good."

"She's not going to die?" Karen asked.

He shook his head.

"Can I kiss you?" She didn't wait for an answer.

Dr. Cook stopped at a light box to show us the films. The mass was right on the surface with no brain around it. The news was, it was a tumor.

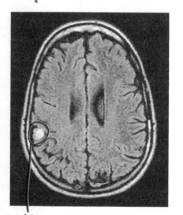

My MRI

Not an aneurysm. Not a cyst. "What about the fluid?" I asked.

"Someone told you there was fluid?" There was no fluid. I glanced at Karen. "Your tumor is acting *benignly*." It had probably been there at least four years, pressing on the brain, causing the seizures. Of course, it would have to come out—he segued right into the operation.

After all the years of buildup, the dreaded brain surgery didn't sound that bad. It sounded comparable, the way he described it, to popping a zit. He would make a little incision, just big enough to insert the foot of a little saw, then zip, zip, zip—out came a piece of skull, not much bigger than the tumor itself, and once the skull was gone—pop!—the brain pressure itself would squeeze the tumor out. Or if he needed to—pluck!—he'd grab it off the surface. Skull goes back on—zoom, zoom, zoom—with titanium plates, which—since everybody asks—do not set off airport metal detectors. Any other questions?

I had a million questions—I settled on one: Can I go on vacation? My mother's bags had been packed for a week.

"France, is it?" (Dr. Hershorin must have told him.) "I don't see why not." We continued down the hall to his office. All of a sudden, I realized how lucky I really was.

Dr. Cook did the same neuro exam Dr. Hershorin had done. And he answered all our questions: I didn't need to change my diet, didn't need to cut out caffeine. I could keep biking, keep up all my normal activities, except, as I must have been told, driving. No driving for six months from the date of a reported seizure.

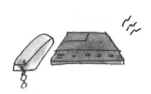

Hello. You've reached the office of Suzy Becker. I'm out RUNNING errands; I expect to be back in 2-3 days. If you'd like to leave a message...

"How are you doing with the medication?"

"I'm not . . . taking the medication," I confessed.

"You might want to start, so you can get back to driving. The state doesn't make any exceptions, whether your seizures are in the middle of the night or only when you're standing on your head." He laced his fingers on top of my folder. "Now, when shall we schedule the surgery?"

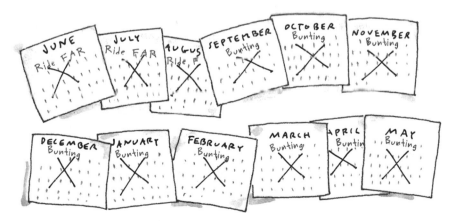

"Next summer." He laughed. I wasn't kidding.

"If I implied it wasn't urgent, I didn't mean it was optional."

"After Christmas."

"You should just come home and get it over with."

"How long before I can get back on my bike?"

Recovery Clock

"How many miles?"

"Fifty."

"Three weeks."

"But, Doctor, I don't know how to ride a bike."

Dr. Cook and Karen groaned.

3 weeks

That *would* give me enough time to train for Ride FAR. . . . They were both staring at me, waiting. *This requires a little more deliberation than buying a TV—more like buying a car. Maybe I could take a night to think it over.* . . . I stared back.

He handed me the films. "Have the desk make an appointment the week you get back, and we'll schedule it then."

My driving ban lasted all of four hours. Karen wasn't used to being the designated driver. On the trip to Dairy Queen (our dinner that night), Karen (1) didn't yield, (2) didn't slow at the flasher at Five Corners (site of the most accidents in the area), and (3) came to a complete stop at a random intersection—no stop signs or lights—a few blocks later.

"I may not make it to surgery," I said, once we'd pulled safely into the parking lot.

She handed me the keys. "You can drive home, but you have to promise not to drive when you're sleep-deprived or if you have a lot* on your mind.

The next morning I called Laura's father, mostly to find out if I would get busted for the driving. "Did they find something?" he asked. I forgot he was back in the pre-test days. I filled him in. "Any chance you can get your films to Laura before you go away? I'd like to have a look at them." *Any chance your opinion will be worse than the one I've got?* I dropped them off at Laura's on my way to the airport.

---

*A small tumor doesn't count.

MY MOTHER'S 71ˢᵗ BIRTHDAY

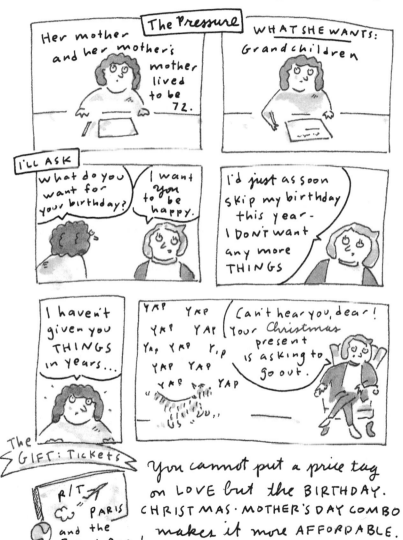

The Pressure

Her mother and her mother's mother lived to be 72.

WHAT SHE WANTS: Grandchildren

I'LL ASK

What do you want for your birthday?

I want *you* to be happy.

I'd just as soon skip my birthday this year — I DON'T want any more THINGS

I haven't given you THINGS in years...

YAP YAP YAP YAP YAP YAP YAP YAP YAP YAP YAP YAP

Can't hear you, dear! Your *Christmas* present is asking to go out.

The GIFT: Tickets

RITA PARIS and the French Open!

You cannot put a price tag on LOVE *but* the BIRTHDAY·CHRISTMAS·MOTHER'S DAY COMBO *makes* it more AFFORDABLE.

The Almost PERFECT GIFT

If I had to tell my mother I had a brain tumor, Paris was the best of all possible places. But I decided to wait until after the French Open. That gave her one half of the week not ruined by the news, and the other half to get used to it.

I took my first Neurontin pill on the plane and checked left to see if my mother had noticed. She was watching the movie, wearing her plane clothes—a matching sweatsuit my sister Robin had painted. I felt a pang of premature nostalgia.

THE THINGS I'LL MISS ABOUT MY MOTHER
(a partial listing)

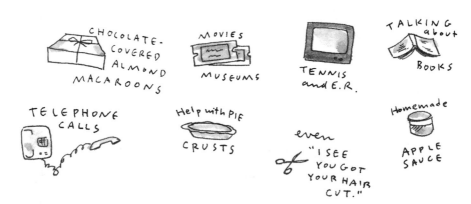

CHOCOLATE-COVERED ALMOND MACAROONS

MOVIES

MUSEUMS

TENNIS and E.R.

TALKING about BOOKS

TELEPHONE CALLS

Help with PIE CRUSTS

even "I SEE YOU GOT YOUR HAIR CUT."

Homemade APPLE SAUCE

Our ★★ hotel was much worse than Karen and I had hoped. The specially requested courtyard-facing room opened on to clotheslines and courtyard noise. I abandoned Karen and my bags and went next door to get my mother's reaction over with. Her windows were wide open, and she was happily unpacking. The hotel was much better than she had feared.

The weather was perfect for the Open. We packed a picnic and sat through four matches; my mother stood up once to stretch her legs. I watched her record all the results in her program, wishing the day would never end.

When we got back to our room, Karen reorganized her camera bag on her side of the bed, and I lay down to come up with a plan.

Telling

WHO: My mother

WHAT: (Tumor. Skip and come back to.)

WHEN: First thing, get up and get it over with, leaving room
    for an afternoon excursion or dinner to resurrect what
    was left of the day.

WHERE: Her room (privacy for potential crying).

HOW: Breakfast in bed.

WHAT: . . .

I rejected Karen's offer to role-play. Playing myself, I've discovered, is harder than being myself.

"Breakfast in bed!" I knocked loudly. I had two coffees, two almond croissants, and the *International Herald Tribune*. She came to the door in her pajamas. "Suzy, this is too much! You've done too much already—" I had not anticipated this part—the feeling I was setting her up for more of a fall. I set the breakfast down on the window ledge. *Before or after breakfast?*   Ruin her appetite or make her sick?

"Where's Karen?" she asked.

"She wanted us to have some time alone." She perked up. I was making it worse. I had to say it. Before breakfast. "Mommy, the day before we left, I found out I have a mass"—I couldn't say *tumor*—"in my head." I told her about the seizures, the testing, and the surgery, leaning heavily on Dr. Cook's good news–bad news technique.

She asked one question. "Is there a name for what you have, the mass in your head?"

I still couldn't say it. "It's on the left parietal lobe." I showed her. "This part above my ear."

She gathered my head to her chest and held it there. "Oh, Suzy." I couldn't tell if she was crying. "I know you, I know you'll—somehow you'll get through this." She didn't bring it up again. Months later, she told me she never slept another night in Paris.

Karen and I had two days alone together at the end of the trip. The morning of the first day, the Metro went on strike. We crammed onto a bus. After sitting in standstill traffic for half an hour, we got off and walked to Père-Lachaise cemetery.

I reeked of B.O., not mine—the shoulder of my last clean shirt had been wedged under the arm of the man holding on to the rail above me. At the cemetery entrance, Karen headed toward Abélard and Héloïse's graves, and I ran for the line of people waiting to fill up their watering cans. After I doused my shoulder, I found a bench and waited for Karen.

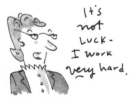

My shoulder dried in the sun. What luck! Some people get defensive about their good luck. I get defensive about my bad luck. I dreaded telling people about my head; I could hear them say how unlucky I was, the way they did when my dog got sick. Like I'm Job. They are not taking my good luck into account.

It's not luck- I work very hard.

SOME PEOPLE

If you're not willing to consider yourself unlucky and leave it at that, then you're bound to ask why. . . .

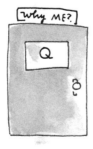

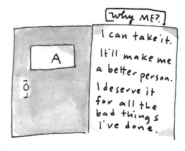

You're better off conceding. Some questions are best left unanswered.

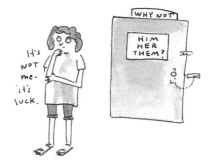

I checked my shoulder—I now had a full-fledged shoulder-smelling tic—and went back to thinking. *I wonder how much of my head they'll shave. . . . I forgot to ask whether I'd be able to do other things besides bike. . . . What about the playwriting seminar at the end of June? . . . What about the pelvic ultrasound? What if I have cervical cancer? What if I have only six months to live? What if I have six years, would I still have the brain surgery?*

Thank god, Karen appeared.

The morning we left Paris, Karen rearranged her camera bag one last time; the twenty rolls of film she'd shot went in a plastic bag on top. When we got to airport security, she pulled out the bag, *"Monsieur, s'il vous plaît, c'est très, très sensible!"* The guy nodded in understanding; her accent had passed all through Paris. He took the plastic bag, then dropped it in a box and sent it through the X-ray machine. Karen shrieked.

By the time I got through, Karen was sitting on the floor—her head on her knees, her back against a ticket counter. "Suz, I can't—" She was shaking her head, sobbing. "I can't take this. I am so scared. I don't want to lose you. . . ." I rubbed her neck. "I haven't cried since, since"—the sobbing stopped while she thought—"since that trailer, the MRI." The sobbing started again. I hadn't given it any thought, the way she'd been holding up— it was hard to remember that it wasn't just happening to me. "You wanted to go to duty free." She gave me a little push. "I'm just going to sit here for a while."

I took a picture of her crying from duty free, sure she would laugh at it when this was all over.

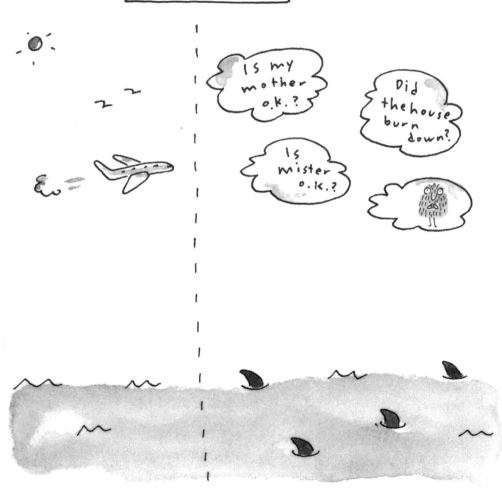

UNCLE!

Everything was fine at home with one minor exception: Mister had scratched his cornea while Laura was taking care of him. The vet's instructions were laid out on the counter next to two books Bruce had left for me from Bill: one from the Brain Tumor Society and the other Audre Lorde's *The Cancer Journals. Cancer* journals?!

I dialed Laura's number on the cordless phone and ran upstairs to throw the books in the corner of my studio. "Does Mister need more eye medicine before bed?" I was ready to hang up—

"My dad wants to talk to you."

"About?"

"He wouldn't tell me. He's around all this weekend."

I called my own dad over the weekend. Both my sisters were visiting him, standing by for the call. I gave him the Dr. Cook good news–bad news, but apparently a lot got lost in this telling.

Meredith called me back. "Dad thinks you have something growing on your skull, a bone chip or something *outside* your brain." She was annoyed. "I'm telling him it's a tumor." I didn't hear back from them after that.

$$\frac{\text{OPTIMISM}}{\text{DENIAL}}$$

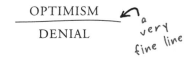 a very fine line

On Monday morning, I postponed calling Dr. Thompson first thing because I had to be able to hand the septic tank cleaner a check in the driveway in order to get the 5 percent discount. Plus, I wouldn't have wanted to miss the septic man saying, "Whatever you're doing, keep up the good work. Your tank looks great!"

Then I didn't call him second thing because I had fifteen cartoons due at the end of the week. And if I didn't make my deadline, I'd have to postpone the surgery, unless Dr. Thompson planned to tell me I was going to die, in which case, I didn't mind a few extra hours before I found out.

I called him after lunch. Dr. Thompson had shown my films to the neuroradiologists at both of Harvard's hospitals, and he had bad news. "It's a tumor."

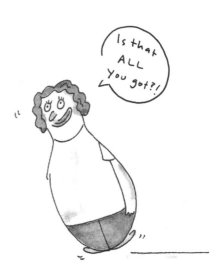

"It's not a meningioma, which I'd hoped. And"—he hesitated— "it's not in a good place."

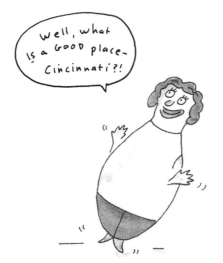

This was the part I hadn't been able to find in my books: "A lot of functions in the brain are duplicated in other areas; some of the areas don't have assigned functions, which means we aren't really sure what they do. It would be preferable to have a tumor in one of those areas, say the front of the brain. Your tumor is in the area that controls

your upper right side mobility. And
there is no duplication of that motor
control anywhere else in the brain.

"You have to understand, this is
brain surgery. Simply exposing the
area to the air . . .

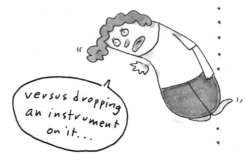

. . . is going to alter it. You should be prepared
to lose some sensation, some fine motor control.

"Did your doctor discuss whether you'd be awake during the surgery?"

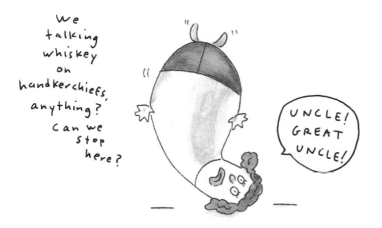

"If it were my family"—and he
considered me family—"there are
only two places to go for this kind of
surgery: Mass General or Brigham
and Women's." He had placed calls
to the top neurosurgeons at both
and was waiting to hear back.

I must have thanked Dr.
Thompson before I hung up the
phone and headed upstairs to the

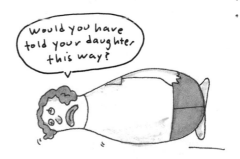

bathroom to study my right side in the mirror. Eyebrow. Eye. Cheek. Nose. Ear. Lips. I smiled. Shoulder. Breast. Arm. Hand. My drawing hand.

The face, not the hand, bothered me most. The first thing people see. The public display of deformity. *How do you prepare?*

Laura called later that afternoon. I ran my assessment by her; she agreed, the face was worse. "You can always draw with your left hand. The drawings are all in your head, not your hand." Those *used* to be my thoughts exactly.

"So if I have to draw with my left hand, will you switch in solidarity?"

"But I wouldn't have a reason."

"Oh, you mean, I could use the brain surgery as a disclaimer."

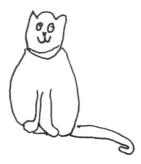

This drawing was created by artist Suzy Becker with the use of her left hand after brain surgery left her partially paralyzed.

Her father called back late that night. He had just finished talking with John Finn, a "prince among men." There were no guarantees that Dr. Finn would do the surgery, but he would meet with me. His patient coordinator had me down for the following Tuesday, 8 A.M.

It had been five weeks since the Bunting-acceptance seizure. There had been no change in my symptoms, no seizures or anything, but now everyone had me convinced I was sick. Part of me wanted to take to my bed. The rest of me redoubled my efforts at feeling normal.

The night before my appointment with Dr. Finn, I tucked Bill's Brain Tumor Society book in my bag so Karen and I could cram for the appointment. I really wanted Dr. Finn to do the surgery—it was the Harvard affiliation, my trust in Dr. Thompson, and the rust-stained toilet bowls alternative.

We opened the book to Chapter 1: "Overview of Brain Tumors." The third section began, "Brain tumors are generally described as 'a cancer.'" That would explain *The Cancer Journals*. Up until then—it probably sounds strange—the possibility of brain cancer had not registered with either one of us.

That was enough reading for me. I rewrote my list of questions for Dr. Finn more legibly and went to bed.

We were Dr. Finn's first appointment. When he stepped through the door, Karen and I reflexively rose. He was shorter than I'd imagined and more humble, inverting all my correlations between height, professional status, and arrogance. He had my vote before we sat down.

At fifty-something, Dr. Finn's face had been shaped by concern and laughter. He never spoke about himself unless we asked, and his time was so valuable, we hardly ever asked. Here are two years' worth of ac-cumulated answers: His Ph.D. is in art history. He *is* the John Finn who is married to a legislator with four kids, all grown. (Karen had heard of his wife.) He is *not* the John Finn who chases storms in his free time (the one Bruce found on the Internet).

> The source of more worry lines as I approach 40

> At age fifty, every man has the face he deserves.
>
> —GEORGE ORWELL

After he did the neurological exam, Dr. Finn put my films up on the light box. I noticed his hands. I had liked Dr. Cook's, but Dr. Finn's were smaller and less manicured, which put me more at ease somehow. In the films Dr. Finn showed us, the tumor didn't appear to be right on the sur-face. A thin layer of brain tissue covered it.

Dr. Finn explained the surgery in detail. He would be operating in the brand-new Magnetic Resonance Therapy Suite, located in the basement—*how Frankensteinian!*—of the hospital. I would be "awake"—by that he meant able to give him feedback—but I would have an anesthesiologist by my side the entire time to make sure I wasn't feeling any pain. Using the MRI technology, he could see that the tumor was completely removed while the skull was still open. . . . At that point, I decided to tune in to a weight-control meeting going on across the hall.

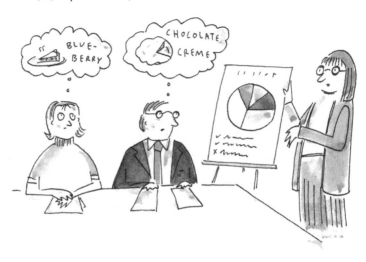

Dr. Finn came back into focus. "Do you have any questions?" I reevaluated my list:

What kind of a brain tumor is it? *Not known per Brain Tumor book.*
Is it malignant? *Ditto.*
Is the medication necessary? Makes me dizzy and tired. *Too whiny.*
Is it possible that the seizures are causing the tumor and not the other way around? *Sounds kooky.*
Could the tumor be affecting my vision? *Or could it be that I*
Recovery?   *haven't seen an eye doctor in eight years?*

Recovery Clock

1 week

"I was curious about the recovery time."
"About a week."
There was one other thing . . .

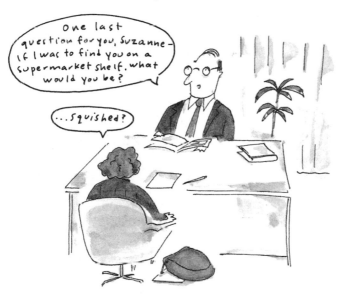

Ask him! "I feel funny asking this." *Especially of some-one with so little.* "I was wondering about my hair." He smiled. "We'll take the minimum. A patch yay big—" The nurses were beeping him; we'd run over. He looked at me. "I was wondering if *you* might answer a question for me—to give me a little better sense of you." I couldn't remember the last time I was so nervous; it felt like an audition. "What three things are most important to you?"

I've learned not to trust my brain in these situations.

MY LAST *Real* JOB INTERVIEW
(Spring of Senior Year)

One last question for you, Suzanne— If I was to find you on a supermarket shelf, what would you be?

...squished?

I wanted to sound like a princess among women, worthy of a prince among men. They were beeping him again. "Making people laugh. Making a difference. My friends and family." *Christ, that's a telephone plan, not an answer. Anybody could have come up with those three things and, oh god, I should have said Karen—*

He handed each of us his card and said, "Why don't you stop and see Katondra on your way out? She'll schedule the surgery."

We hurried down the hall to claim our prize.

Katondra was perfect for her job: bossy and big-hearted. Laughter among medical office personnel had started to make me feel cranky and invisible, but Katondra had this booming laugh that made me hope someone would say something funny. She was on the phone, holding. "Suzy Becker, come over here, I can talk to you." She looked down at her book and back up at me. "I can fit you in a week from Friday."

As in ten days from today? "I was thinking of something a little later . . . y'know, like—" *Never.* Keep the prize.

She rolled her eyes. "Suzy, Suzy, I'm trying to get you home for the Fourth of July."

"Suz?" Karen looked at me.

"Okay."

Done. Katondra wrote me in the book. She put whoever she was holding for on hold and scheduled my pre-admit testing. "You report here, downstairs, at six A.M. on the twenty-fifth." She underlined the A.M. and handed us the paper with all my appointments.

"Should I give blood?" *Isn't that what people do before surgery?*

"Nope, not necessary. There's not much blood in the brain. No aspirin, nothing that has aspirin in it between now and then. No food or drink after midnight the night before." She smiled at me. "You're going to be fine."

Hey, what about a nonsurgical opinion?

The FLIGHT of the CONDOR

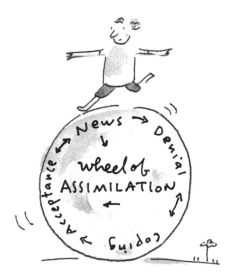

For someone who had never had to cope with anything worse than stitches, I thought I had done a pretty good job maintaining equilibrium during the diagnostic phase. But now I realized that my sense of equilibrium had been propped up by an artificially high level of ignorance on everybody else's part. I had put off telling friends, editors, Ride FAR people, etc., by telling myself (and Karen) that there simply wasn't enough to tell.

Now we had all the information, and I *had* to start telling. Brain surgery isn't one of those things you casually allude to later. "Are you sure? I thought I'd mentioned it. . . ."

TELLING Berkeley JANE

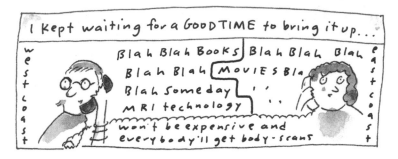

I kept waiting for a GOOD TIME to bring it up...

west coast / east coast

Blah Blah BOOKS Blah Blah Blah
Blah Blah MOVIES Bla
Blah Someday
MRI technology
won't be expensive and everybody'll get body-scans

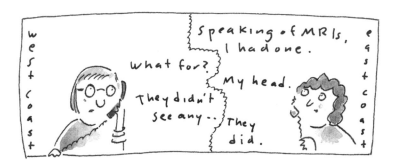

west coast / east coast

Speaking of MRIs, I had one.
What for?
My head.
They didn't see any --
They did.

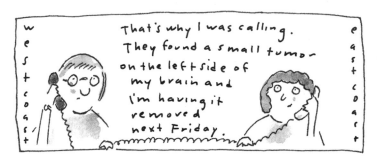

west coast / east coast

That's why I was calling. They found a small tumor on the left side of my brain and I'm having it removed next Friday.

She was going to be at a friend's for the weekend. Assuming all went well, someone would leave a message on the friend's machine: The CONDOR HAS LANDED.

Each time I told someone, I tried to remember how it was hearing it for the first time. But to me, the more I said it, the less real it sounded, the opposite of the way telling a lie over and over can make it seem true.

Within a day, my brain tumor became gossip; I got a condolence call from somebody I hardly knew.

I panicked at the loss of control and called my therapist. She was easy to tell, either because she is a therapist and she wouldn't want me to worry about her feelings, or because her husband had had a tumor. (News to me.) It was in his pituitary, like Bill's. When she told me, I knew enough by then to interject, "They remove those through the nose."

All of my telling, she helped me see, was at cross-purposes with my goal of feeling healthy and preparing for surgery. "Have you thought about a Web site?"

I didn't have one; I would need someone else to put it up—and it was not how I had envisioned my launch. I decided to make a list of calls and give it to Karen or my sisters. There were people I could leave off the list: not everyone *had* to know, such as people I didn't want second-guessing my brain, wondering if they'd taken too much off the top. Ride FAR people. And editors. Humor is a very subjective business.

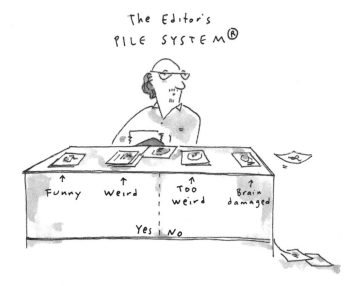

FINDINGS ON INTERCESSORY PRAYER
Out of 990 subjects in a Kansas coronary care unit, half were prayed for by regular churchgoers and half were not. None were told about the intervention so their hopes and beliefs would not affect outcome. A 10 percent better outcome was reported for the prayed-for group.

—*ABSTRACT ARCHIVES OF INTERNAL MEDICINE*

Once I let go—let other people do the telling—it didn't feel like I'd lost anything. The more people knew, the merrier. I could use all the praying and chanting and drumming, visualizing, lighting candles, and finding of four-leaf clovers I could get.

On June 20, 1999, the Monday before my surgery, I heard from Katondra. They needed to move the surgery back a week. *Isn't that move up, since last Friday's already gone by?* There was a patient who wouldn't make it unless Dr. Finn operated.

I understood. *But what about my dad's flight? What about how Meredith and Bruce took the day off? All the people who are praying for the wrong day? Who's going to take care of Mister? The condor landing? And what about the Fourth of July you promised me—me and Karen lying on our backs on a boat, watching the fireworks—the only scrap of a visualization I've ever had? When I suggested scheduling the surgery a little later, it was a bad idea, but now, now that I'm ready to go through with it . . .*

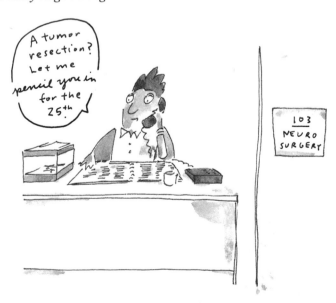

The preadmission schedule didn't change. Karen dropped me at the hospital doors and went to park the car. I signed in and slouched in my chair. Any novelty about the place had worn off. I was bored by the forms. Blasé about the bloodletting. All my senses dulled down. No listening in. No eyeballing the sick people. No second-sniffing unfamiliar smells. The hospital was the one remaining setting I didn't consider *myself* sick in; I was a healthy person with an aberration. ⟶

ME: A Perfect 12

CARDIAC EXERCISE TOLERANCE

1 EATING, GETTING DRESSED, WORKING AT A DESK
2 SHOWERING, WALKING DOWN EIGHT STEPS
3 WALKING ON A FLAT SURFACE FOR ONE OR TWO BLOCKS
4 RAKING LEAVES, WEEDING, OR PUSHING A POWER MOWER
5 WALKING 4 MILES PER HOUR, SOCIAL DANCING, WASHING A CAR
6 NINE HOLES OF GOLF CARRYING CLUBS, HEAVY CARPENTRY, USING PUSH MOWER
7 DIGGING, SPADING SOIL, SINGLES TENNIS, CARRYING 60 POUNDS
8 MOVING HEAVY FURNITURE, JOGGING SLOWLY, RAPIDLY CLIMBING STAIRS, CARRYING 20 POUNDS UPSTAIRS
9 BICYCLING AT A MODERATE PACE, SAWING WOOD, SLOW JUMPING ROPE
10 BRISK SWIMMING, BICYCLING UPHILL, WALKING BRISKLY UPHILL, JOGGING 6 MPH
11 CROSS-COUNTRY SKIING, FULL-COURT BASKETBALL
12 RUNNING CONTINUOUSLY AT 8 MPH

I was deemed fit to go under the knife, and the preadmit nurse was ready to get rid of us, unless we had any questions. "Will I be recovering on the cancer floor?" (The C-word would require some extra advance preparation of my parents or some major on-site distractions.)

"He has you down for four to five hours in the operating room; then you'll be admitted to neuro-ICU. You'll spend at least a day there. They have one nurse for each patient; they have to watch very carefully for any signs of bleeding, infection, or seizure activity. Your visiting hours are unrestricted, but you're allowed only one"—she held up one finger—"visitor at a time. After that, they'll move you to the tenth floor."

I had another question, sprung from my keen medical intuition—the kind to ask someone I would never be seeing again. "After they take the tumor out, do they put something back in to take up the extra space, the pressure—" My thinking, my worry was that the extra pressure was necessary for the optimal functioning of my brain or, conversely, without it my brain would go slack.

She acted as if it were a reasonable question. "The pressure is causing the seizures. Once the tumor is removed, the seizures should go away and your brain will fill in the space itself."

One last logistical question: "Do the rooms have modems?"

I'd actually made her laugh. "A hospital is a place to recuperate, not work." She was done with us; she wished me good luck with frightening sincerity.

The anesthesiologist's stand-in saw us next. Resident Dr. Heinemann was perfectly cast for his part: immaculately groomed, soft-spoken, with a slight German accent. His first few sentences lulled me into a state of blanket acceptance.

". . . and then you'll fall fast asleep."

"Asleep?" I interrupted, "I'm supposed to be awake!"

"That's not what it says here." He flashed the clipboard at me, then went to check the paperwork before he explained any further.

What else *does it say or not say there?* Karen was relieved. "Suz, imagine if they had put you out. . . ."

The idea of being asleep now scared me more than being awake ever had—the notion of giving up my power of observation, my power to grab the instruments (or the doctor by the necktie) if things started going awry . . .

Dr. Heinemann couldn't find anybody to verify the "awake" part of my surgery, but our conviction persuaded him to tell us about it anyway. "Awake surgery is also known as conscious sedation," he explained. I would feel some things: hot and cold, pressure on my head, but the brain itself doesn't feel pain.

BILATERAL CONFUSION (a.k.a. wrong site surgery and symmetry failure): In November 1995, a doctor at Sloan-Kettering performed brain surgery on the wrong hemisphere of his patient's brain.

"What about the noise, the saw?" I asked, since there was no pain to worry about. "It's so close to my ear." I was picturing a chain saw.

"The drill is louder. But both will sound like they're in some distant land. And the drugs are amnestics; they'll help you forget everything after it's over."

The Drill

The first night, Dr. Heinemann went on, the ICU nurse would wake me up every fifteen minutes. And he told me to expect a migraine for the first forty-eight hours. I'd never had a migraine, so I didn't know what to expect, and I didn't care to imagine. I interrupted instead, exaggerating my enunciation, "Dr. Heinemann, your English is very good."

He shook his head. "If you were my sister, I would have made sure Dr. Finn was your surgeon. He's The Guy."

"He's The Man." I nodded. And it's true, he is. I hear it over and over, to this day.

Our last meeting was with Dr. Finn's nurse. It was after 5 P.M., and Karen and I were wiped out, mostly from all the waiting. The nurse handed us a "patient education pamphlet." When she saw me count the six pages of information, she said, "Don't worry, we'll just go over the most important points." There were three: (1) no vomiting (request anti-nausea medication); (2) no bending over; and (3) no straining when moving your bowels, which added up to one Big Message. No intra-cranial pressure (ICP). No brain popping out the hole in your head.

ICP ALERT!

The nurse went over a few studies. The hospital was a teaching and re-search facility and I was being asked to participate, with the disclaimer that my decision would in no way affect the medical care I received. *The way not buying the magazines has never affected my chances of becoming a finalist in the Publishers Clearing House Sweepstakes . . .*

"Do you have any questions?" Last call . . .

I had a question—more of a second thought, really.

"I was nervous—I think I was trying to impress Dr. Finn, um, when he asked me about the three most important things, and, the more I've thought about it—none of those things really depended on my right side. I think it's one of those things you, I, take for granted, I mean, normally

I don't think someone would say, 'My right side,' so it might not have seemed like a big deal, throw my upper right side away, but it is, would be—"

"I'll let Dr. Finn know, unless, did you want to tell him yourself?"

I shook my head.

"Dr. Finn has seen your books, Suzy. He understands the importance of your right side. If removing the tumor were going to diminish the quality of your life, your work, I know him—he'd be more likely to leave a piece of it in and figure out some other way to deal with it."

That was all the reassurance I needed. *Almost.* "I know you can't tell what kind of tumor I have until you get the biopsy results, but—Karen and I were reading the Brain Tumor Society book, and a lot of the people had tumors that weren't 'cancerous,' except they grew back. Sometimes within a few months. Is that—what are the chances of *that* happening?"

"We'll need the biopsy." Her face was apologetic. "Let's just get you through the surgery; then in three or four weeks, when we have all the information, we'll sit down and go over your treatment plan"—*TREAT-MENT PLAN?!*—"whether you'll need additional radiation in that spot or chemotherapy." Her voice sounded like it was coming from the end of a very long tunnel. It was the first time anyone had uttered the words *treatment plan, radiation,* or *chemotherapy.*

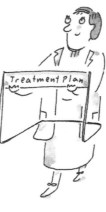

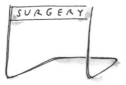

I asked Karen, once we were in the hall, for confirmation. "Had you heard, has anyone ever said anything about a treatment plan before?"

She put an arm around my shoulders and pulled me close while we walked. "No, sweetie."

I read the patient pamphlet before bed that night. I already knew everything in it. I felt prepared.

TERRY GROSS: But, it turns out, in some fairly significant ways, you weren't prepared at all. . . .

ME: Don't give away the rest of the story.

TG: Did you keep that patient education pamphlet?

ME: I've reread it a dozen times. And I've looked at my notes from that day to see if there was something I missed.

TG: What about a nonsurgical opinion?

ME: Next time. I don't know. . . . I mean, I hope there is no next time. I remember thinking at some point, post-Cook, pre-Finn, "Of course, a surgeon recommends surgery." But with the trip to France—or maybe the neurologist's vacation—everything, the timeline got compressed. "Go directly to the neurosurgeon, do not pass Go!" Five days before surgery, I wasn't thinking about a nonsurgical opinion.

And it wasn't just the neurosurgeons; all the neuroradiologists said the same thing.

TG: I would think writing this next part, essentially reliving the operating-room scenes, must have been difficult. I presume that's why we're talking now. What about some of your other forms of procrastination—

ME: You mean the movie?

TG: Starring?

ME: Starring Winona Ryder, her comeback from the shoplifting thing. And you, if you want, as yourself.

GETTING MY
DUCKS in a ROW

Documents

I found a new lawyer to update my will. I didn't need the expensive lawyer to FIND Amy (old partner) and REPLACE with Karen (new partner) throughout the document, but I did need to deal with my house. I wanted to will it to Robin. Karen didn't need a third house, and everybody else in my family was covered.

"Hey, Rob," I asked her over the phone, "if I died, would you want the house?"

"Do I have to take Mister with it?"

"Ha, ha, ha." *Meredith would take Mister . . . or she'd find him a good home.*

Robin was quiet for a second, "I love it, Suz . . . but I don't know if I could afford to—I don't know how it would compare with my rent."

"I'm leaving you some money."

She started crying. "I'm sorry. Of course . . . I was just—there's so much of *you* there, and all the Christmases—and if that was all that was left—oh. I'm embarrassed . . . Can we forget the first part of the conversation?"

"Yep. Now don't get your hopes up or anything—no disappointment if I don't die."

The lawyer made all the changes within a few days, and I went to his office to sign my new will. Two tellers from the bank downstairs served as witnesses. I followed him back up to his office and watched him slip his fountain pen back in the inside pocket of his suit jacket before I realized we were done. "Good luck," he said. I was just about to thank him. "And would you mind dropping a check in the mail *before* the operation?"

Hair

I had made an appointment to get my hair cut Thursday, formerly known as the day before my surgery. It could be likened to landscaping the yard before digging up the septic system, but my hair was already overdue, and it would be a long time before I let someone near it with a comb or scissors again.

This was only my second time with this stylist. We hadn't found our conversational groove. "Any plans for the Fourth of July?" she asked.

That's a new one, let's see. . . . None of my answers to "How are you?" worked. "Wow! Is that next weekend already?" I was aiming for "Summer's really flying by."

"You going away? Staying in town?"

"Staying."

"Going to the fireworks?" She had stopped cutting and was waiting for my answer in the mirror.

Okay, if you must know: "Nope. Going to have brain surgery, actually."

She went back to cutting. "I'm really good at wigs if you need any help with that—I took one of my other clients shopping. We had a lot of fun."

It was a kind offer, I acknowledged, silently hoping I'd never have to take her up on it. She charged me half for the haircut.

Visitors

My mother wanted to be at the hospital the morning of my surgery to see me, her daughter, off to the operating room, but I had set my limit at three people: Meredith, Karen, and Karen's best friend, Patty. The more people, the bigger deal. Plus, I couldn't worry about my mother's worrying, not that morning. MY MOTHER'S WORRY → ME WORRY (ABOUT HER + VICARIOUSLY ABOUT MYSELF).

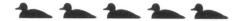

Robin helped me solve part of the problem by asking my mother to drive her to the hospital so she wouldn't get lost. My mother (who will make sure the story of how Robin got lost at Expo 1967 is never forgotten) agreed, so the two of them wouldn't be arriving until the afternoon. This meant the next time I saw my mother, I'd be in the ICU. *I better let her know that.*

I made plans to see her for dinner. During the course of the conversation, she asked whether I'd have my own private room. "Well, yes." *I could not have come up with a better spin myself.* "I'll have my own private room, with my own private nurse, and it's all covered by my insurance. I'm in what they call neurointensive care after the surgery, not because I'm critically ill—they have to be extra careful about infection with brain surgery."

It seemed to go over. After we said good-bye, I caught myself thinking, *And that was the last time I ever saw my mother. . . . Silly thought.* I repeated it over and over, emphasizing a different word each time. And that *was,* and that was *the,* and that was the *last . . .*

Work

I sent the ten finished cartoons off to my editor. That batch would see me through September 15. *Fannie Farmer's weekly columns appeared for months after she died.* Another dead thought. *Healthy. Very healthy.*

That was it, my last duck. Done. I was all set for surgery, and I still had a whole week to go. *There must be something I'm forgetting.*

Bruce called. "Remember *not* to tape the healing statements to your clothes today; your surgery has been rescheduled for *next* Friday."

The statements appeared in the book he'd given me, *Prepare for Surgery, Heal Faster,* along with a "don't hold me responsible, unless it's helpful" disclaimer. I didn't hold him responsible until I got to page six; then I *had* to call him and make him listen to me read out loud:

Healing Statements for Surgery

Patient's Name *Suzy Becker*

(Give this page to your surgeon and another to your anesthesiologist. Tape a third page to your hospital gown so it is visible as you go into surgery.)

As I am going under the anesthesia, please say:

#1 "Following the operation, you will feel comfortable and you will heal very well." (Repeat 5 times.)

After saying the statements, please put on my earphones and start my tape player.

Toward the end of surgery, remove my earphones. Say:

#2 "Your operation has gone very well." (Repeat 5 times.)

#3 "Following this operation, you will be hungry for *crème brûlée* **"**

   "You will be thirsty and you will urinate easily." (Repeat 5 times.)

#4 "Following this operation (fill in your surgeon's recommendations for recovery)

_____

_____." (Repeat 5 times.)

I am allergic to anesthesias and medications: *Sulfa drugs*

The medications and the dosages I am taking are: *Neurontin 300mg*

The book was still sitting where I'd chucked it, on top of *The Cancer Journals*. The unfunny part of his reminder was (I had to remind myself), I had prepared to go *to* surgery, not through surgery. I had effectively avoided thinking about the surgery itself altogether. But as luck would have it, I still had a week. I opened the book to see if I could cherry-pick a few choice principles and techniques to complement my own.

STEP ONE: THE RELAXATION PROCESS. Guided visualization.

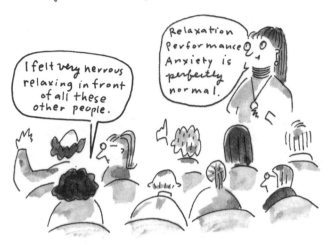

Skip.

STEP TWO: VISUALIZE YOUR HEALING. "Before and after your operation, ask the part of your body that is healing what comforting feeling you
can give it." Example: One woman asked her uterus and it told her to stop
hating it. When she filled it with love, she got out of the hospital two days
early. Another example: A woman had to give her gallbladder "waves of
love" and a little bit of chocolate (not allowed on gallbladder diet). Her attacks disappeared, and her surgery was canceled.

It was worth a try. I asked my brain what I could give it. "I *KNEW*
YOU WERE GOING TO ASK ME THAT."

"Okay, so, you're smarter than a uterus. C'mon, there must be something—don't make me beg—tell me what you want."

"I WANT THE TUMOR."

Great. What does it say in the book about that? "You can't have the
tumor. The doctor has already decided to remove the tumor. Try to think
of something else. Chocolate?"

"THE TUMOR STAYS."

"You must be feeling very afraid right now. No one likes change. Maybe you're worried that the tumor is an important source of something, your creativity, your proper pressure, maybe it's a transmitter from another planet. Let's think about the bigger picture for a minute—if the tumor stays, I could go. Hmm? Think about what that would mean; you don't really want that." *You're talking to your brain like it's a three-year-old.*

I decided the book wasn't meant for brain surgery, and I went back to the Brain Tumor Society book to see if I could find any patients' accounts of the surgery itself. The editor of the book, I noted, had also had a pituitary tumor.

I wanted to read something by someone with a *real* tumor, one that came out the skull, not the nose, with some odds of being malignant.

I couldn't find anything, and the harder I looked, the more I knew I needed to hear what awake brain surgery was like from someone who had had it. Not a resident or a surgeon. I wanted someone who *really* knew to tell me I was going to make it through this part okay. I needed that kind of faith more than prayers right now.

The book listed a number for a brain tumor support group based in Boston. It wasn't like I had anything against support groups.

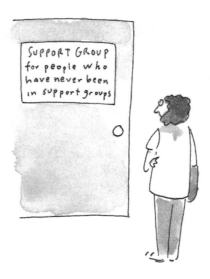

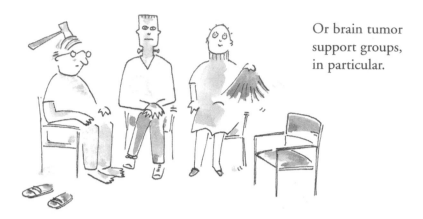

Or brain tumor support groups, in particular.

Bruce said he would call for me. The group met alternate Wednesdays. And this Wednesday?

"Sorry, Suz, no meeting."

I gave up on the idea. Maybe if I had called myself, I would've asked or they would've offered to hook me up with one of the members. And then, when I got out of surgery, I would've had someone to talk to. . . . Another thing I'd do differently next time.

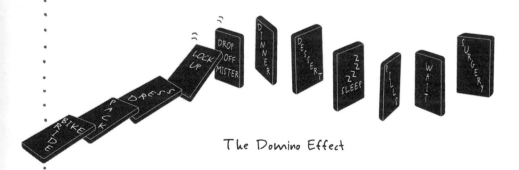

The Domino Effect

The afternoon before my surgery, I had visualized going on a long bike ride with Meredith, but somebody with more clout had visualized rain. It was dark and teeming. We went on a short ride anyway, to kill some time. After hot showers, we sat on the couch in front of the fireplace, and I told her everything, every last thing I was afraid of.

"It feels good to say it out loud," I ended, and we laughed at the "feeling good" since we were bawling. *There weren't* that *many things on my list.* Being alone was the biggest. It was my biggest fear about dying, too. Of course, after I'd admitted that, it was hard to get Meredith to leave me alone so I could pack.

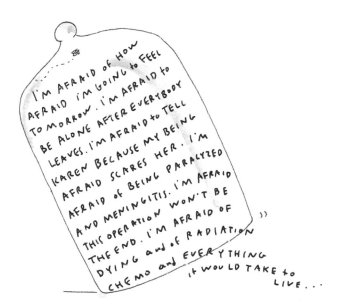

Karen honked twice in the driveway. I turned on the outside lights and pulled the door shut with a slam—a measure of the humidity, not of my resolve. I drove us up to the North Shore—away from Boston, away from the hospital—to drop Mister off and go out for dinner. *I still have the whole night.*

We were sitting in our favorite spot—a funny corner made of two windows, no wall, that juts out over a little harbor—at our favorite restaurant. After we'd ordered, we set gifts out on the table. The server put our salads off to the side. "Somebody having a birthday?"

[handwritten margin note: ? when do you anniversarize? FIRST date? FIRST kiss? FIRST sleep-over?]

"No—" We laughed. The real answer sounded dumb. It was our eleven-month anniversary. We had butted heads so often back in the beginning, it was a miracle we made it through the first month. Or the second. So we got in the habit of celebrating each month. The presents weren't usually anything big. I had a pair of dachshund corn holders for Karen.

I picked up Karen's present, and she said, "Suz, I'm really sorry; I wanted to save it for our one-year anniversary." She was crying. The server retreated.

"You *can*." I put the bag down and hugged her. "I'm not going to die. I'm really not." She was wiping her eyes. "Too late, then." I had the bag again. "I'm keeping it." There was a baseball glove inside. My first non-hand-me-down mitt.

I had a new visualization, something to replace my old Fourth of July on-our-backs-on-the-boat fireworks: playing catch on a stretch of the beach, with the two dogs running back and forth . . . *unless I couldn't catch. Wait—no, I'd still be able to catch. I might not be able to throw.*

After dinner, we walked down the street, prolonging the night. I got an ice cream; Karen ordered a decaf espresso with a twist. I watched the summer helper squeeze a wedge of lemon into the miniature paper cup. I couldn't wait to see Karen's reaction. She just drank it.

The drive back was quiet. Shorter somehow. We pulled into the gravel driveway just before midnight. I got out of the driver's seat and just stood by the car door. I thought I might feel an urge to run or walk around the block. *No.* I felt calm, compliant. I felt like going in and getting it over with, taking my pill and going to bed.

Karen set the alarm for five-something. It wasn't until she reached for the light that I felt an urge. "I'm going to read for a while."

"You should rest for tomorrow," she said.

"I can rest while I'm in the hospital." I climbed down from the loft and took out the John Irving book I'd bought for my convalescence. Karen had covered her head with the pillow by the time I climbed back up. I read the first three chapters before giving in. I put Karen's head back on top of her pillow, wove my arm under her arm, over her stomach, and slept.

ENGINE, ENGINE NUMBER 9

Karen woke first and went downstairs to shower and make her coffee. I stayed up in the loft. The alarm clock blinked 5:30. All of Karen's clocks are fast. 5:32. 33. 34. I never know how fast.

"All done! I'll be ready to go in five," she yelled. *Translation: Ten to fifteen.* I climbed down, brushed my teeth without swallowing any toothpaste, got dressed, and took my pills with the minimum of water.

Fifty simple things you can do to avoid surgery (day of):

1. Oversleep
2. Eat 2 inches of toothpaste or a big breakfast
3. Down six glasses of water, OJ, or other liquid
4. . . . .

I strung my ring on my necklace and laid it beside my wallet on my place mat. Then I looked around, a halfhearted search for something to keep us from leaving. "See ya, Moll." I went over to pat Karen's beagle good-bye. Karen held the door, quietly waiting, and we walked out. I felt strangely unencumbered as I walked down the stairs, carrying just a small bag, wearing gym shorts and flip-flops. Not free, stripped.

Patty (Karen's friend) was waiting in the hospital lobby when we walked through the door at 5:55. The admitting office was open, in view, to the left. The gift shop was closed. Patty took out a softball and lobbed it in my direction; the three of us played catch in the deserted lobby until exactly six o'clock. Then ten more tosses. Just two more, ending on a good one.

I handed copies of my living will and health care proxy to the woman at the admissions desk, and she snapped a blue hospital ID bracelet around my wrist.

Admitted. No more paperwork, just a "Be seated" and a concerned smile; then she called the next patient's name.

The office was filling up. I recognized an older woman from the brain tumor clinic. Her wheelchair was parked at an odd angle, left dangling in front of the row of chairs. Her family was talking behind her; she was staring at the floor.

Karen and Patty were talking beside me. I was communing with the older woman; the two of us sitting there about to get brain surgery, no one talking to us—

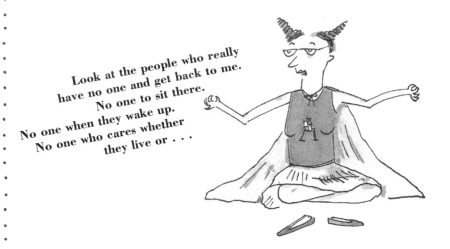

Look at the people who really have no one and get back to me.
No one to sit there.
No one when they wake up.
No one who cares whether they live or . . .

When I am better, I will volunteer in the admissions office—I will sit with people who have no one and hold their hands . . . Maybe I'll go take the woman's hand now, and tell her I know exactly how she feels.

Oh please. Who wants a stranger holding her hand?

My sister Meredith walked in. After she sat down, I could see the admitter pointing the nurse-escort in our direction. I avoided eye contact until she was standing directly in front of me. "Suzy?" Her name was Angela.

Meredith and Patty assumed this was good-bye. "You can come, too— We're going down to the basement waiting area. Just the one bag?" Angela inquired, as if I were boarding a plane.

"Some CDs and my pajamas," I said.

"You can let your friends take your CDs. No music in the suite."

"But Dr. Finn said—"

"Music causes interference with the electronic devices."

Now how am I going to pass the time? Visualization and praying were out. *Alphabet games?*

Angela left us to wait. The second waiting area was decorated with poster-size photographs of the new machinery. If they were meant to be inspirational, they were having the opposite effect. As the on-deck patient, I got the uncomfortable feeling I was about to be operated on by a machine, not by a man.

Patty and Meredith were just finishing flipping them over when Angela came back. "You don't like those? People love them! The new technology is so impressive; it's amazing what they can do!"

ALTERNATIVE ART

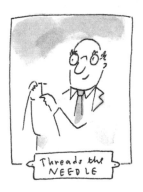

Threads the
NEEDLE

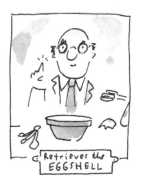

Retrieves the
EGGSHELL

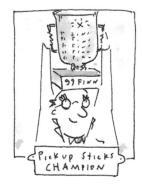

Pickup Sticks
CHAMPION

It was time for Meredith and Patty to go. Karen would've gone, too; this time, I had to ask if it was okay for her to stay. I didn't blame any of them for wanting to leave.

Angela led Karen and me through the double doors. It wasn't anything like I'd pictured. I hadn't expected windows, but the place was dimly lit. The air was thick, not crisp. And the people shuffled by in street clothes, just getting to work, catching up over coffee, like it was any other job.

I got into my johnny.

> In another moment down went Alice . . . never once considering how in the world she was supposed to get out again.
>
> —LEWIS CARROLL, *ALICE IN WONDERLAND*

Angela showed me to a bed with a wraparound curtain. She took one last look at my paperwork, where the shellfish allergy was noted. "Shellfish, I think that's what I'm going to have for lunch today!"

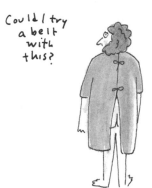

ATTENTION ALL SUITE PERSONNEL:

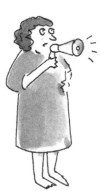

There will be N_O lunch today. You are to STOP acting like this is any other day effective IMMEDIATELY. I AM HAVING BRAIN SURGERY. I repeat: LUNCH CANCELED TODAY. (Sorry to interrupt your coffee.)

"Dr. Finn will be in next," Angela said as she was leaving, which reminded me that I had a card for him in my bag with the CDs. I had considered taping it to my gown.

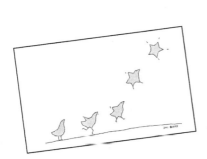
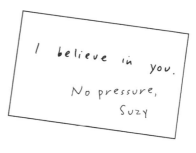

Angela came back; since Karen and I were both authors, she thought we'd like to know that Michael Palmer had been in the week before.

Who? I thought.

"For surgery?" Karen asked.

"Oh, no—he was researching a medical mystery." I appreciated the filler; left on our own, Karen and I sat there in silence. Angela came back one more time to give me the morning lineup: after Dr. Finn, I'd get my IVs, a catheter ("Since you can't be lying there, saying, 'Hey folks, I gotta go to the bathroom'* in the middle of brain surgery"), some pneumatic boots—"not your Nancy Sinatra made-for-walking variety, these keep the blood moving through your legs—" She stopped. Dr. Finn was at the curtain opening.

He pulled up a chair and sat, as if he had nothing more pressing (like changing into his operating clothes) to do. I asked him about the CDs first thing. He could give up one audio channel so they could play my music. He then went over the plan again: once the IVs were set up, the anesthesiologist would give me something to help me relax a little, and then they'd shave my head. The residents would do most of the prep work. "Before we do anything else, we'll do some imaging—the MRIs—so we know exactly where to go in. Then we'll take a little bit of bone out. Then I'll be ready to go in—you'll hear me saying, 'Move your leg, squeeze your hand.' Then, we'll close you up, and get you out of here. . . . Any questions?"

*Bathroom Facts about Me, a.k.a. "The Camel": I can drive Boston–D.C., teach 7a.m.–7p.m. with 0 bathroom stops.

I shook my head.

"Are you okay?"

Avoiding surgery (day of, cont'd.)

4. Have a freak-out in the operating suite

5. Make a run for the doors

6. . . .

I nodded. He cocked his head, trying to meet my eyes. "I'm okay," I said, and handed him the card.

He didn't open it, looked back at me and smiled. "We'll do our best," he said.

The anesthesiologist entered next. Not the real anesthesiologist— another resident. He opened by asking if I'd ever had anesthesia before.

"Novocain," I answered.

"Doesn't count. This is going to be a whole new experience," he said. He was staring at my arms while he said it.

It doesn't matter whether I like him or not. The real anesthesiologist is the one who'll be holding my hand during the operation.

He turned my arms over. "I'm going to set up two lines, a second for backup. We don't have time to replace a line during an awake surgery." He rapped on my left arm while he was explaining.

Maybe he's just nervous. "I have good veins," I said to put him at ease.

More rapping, then the tourniquet. My veins were bulging. I turned to look at Karen; I'm better off not watching.

"First," he said (and I turned back to listen), "the local anesthetic."

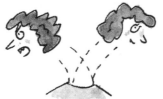

Just
SHUT UP
and
GET IT OVER WITH!

Great.
Thanks so much
for the
heads-up.

DON'T LISTEN to HER!

The needle hovered above the vein. I turned away, and it slipped in. He loosened the tourniquet, rapped, and was ready to go again.

Karen's time must almost be up. . . . I was beaming her good-bye love when he had his first miss . . . and his second, after which he stood up and paced around the bed, talking to himself (I think). "I can't use the right arm because they need it during the surgery. . . ."

Tell Junior to get his professor in here PRONTO!

Junior, unprompted, went to consult with someone on the other side of the curtain. He came back and put the second IV in my right hand, the one the real anesthesiologist was supposed to be holding. "Just for backup," he explained a third time, and started the sedative: Drip. Drip. Drip.

"So, you're an artist!" It was Dr. Finn's head resident Steve. Time for my head shaving. "Dr. Finn showed us your book." Time for Karen to go.

Not a single muscle tensed; it was all okay. Okay to shave my head, okay for Karen to go. Here, kiss me good-bye, and she was gone.

Steve lifted my hair and rubber-banded it on the top of my head. As he shaved my head, I was drifting in and out.

I remember worrying that my body would retain all its fluids and I'd end up like Violet in *Charlie and the Chocolate Factory*. I asked the nurse whether that had ever happened. She just laughed. *Listen,* I silently coached my body parts, *just for today, it's okay to go.*

Angela covered me in a blanket, and I was wheeled through another door. I must have been just outside the mouth of the machine, lying there on my back, but I never raised my head to see it. I never thought to look at anything but the ceiling.

Angela waved the catheter bag—thumbs up—the system was working. Then I was rolled onto my side. This was the position I'd be in the entire time, she explained as she tucked a pillow between my knees. *But, I thought I'd be on my back (no one was ever on their side on* ER*) looking up at my team, giving them feedback. . . .*

The real anesthesiologist was talking to a nurse by the wall. I wondered when he was going to take my hand, join the team, but in the next instant, I was off the team. They covered my head in blankets—surgical sheets?—that blocked the light and trapped my breath. *Hello! If anybody is interested in my feedback—it is 150 degrees in here, my hip and shoulder are throbbing, and we haven't even started.* I would have had to yell to be heard. The anesthesiologist was still talking to the nurse by the wall.

Now he was next to me. "We're going to start with a local anesthetic." I felt a burning under my scalp.

Fingertips tacked something to my head—pinned my head to something—so it wouldn't move.

I was awake, as in aware, not alert. Partially aware—I had no visual information, no mental picture to work with, but I heard everything. The drill, two inches above my left ear, sounded like a dentist's drill. I didn't feel it; not going in, not the slight catch just before it broke through.

Steve was calling for "paddies, more paddies." I felt the pressure of paddies—sponges? no, gauze pads, gauze paddies . . . my brain was bleeding. Someone went out of the room for more paddies. *The brain does* not *bleed.*

"Christ! Dammit!" Steve was swearing, and I was trying to measure his swears, gauge how bad it was.

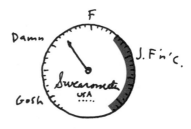

I was starting to feel faint from the loss of blood, or maybe just the suggestion. *Is losing consciousness fainting in this case . . . or dying? I'm not going to die on the operating table. Am I?*

ASK HIM!

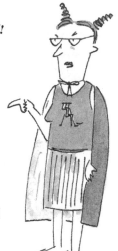

It wasn't a good time to interrupt.

Then don't interrupt! Excuse yourself, say, Pardon, but I can hear every last thing you're saying and . . .

Once the bleeding seemed to be back under control, I spoke for the first time. "Everything okay up there?"

"We're just about ready for Dr. Finn," Steve answered.

"Can I move?"

"What do you want to move?"

Not my head. "My shoulder and hip."

"Go ahead." No matter which way I moved, there was still bone against table. I gave up, and the operation resumed. Someone went to get Dr. Finn.

At this point, if I had understood the explanations correctly, my scalp was sliced open and parted. My skull bone removed. The leathery dura covering the brain had been cut and peeled back, and my innards were exposed.

I tried, but I was incapable of imagining what that *really* looked like.

Dr. Finn was at the table. The anesthesiologist was holding my hand. Steve briefed Dr. Finn on the tumor's location. And Dr. Finn began.

He proceeded slowly, asking for my feedback continuously, "Squeeze your right hand. . . . Move your right leg. . . . Are you okay? . . . You're doing great. . . ."

Updates, based on the images—where the tumor was, where Dr. Finn's instrument was—were broadcast over the audio channel. There was downtime while he waited for new images. Then he went back in.

He asked me to squeeze. Move my leg—"Beautiful! Got it!"
The tumor was out!

There was a pause. Silence. No celebration. Then the intercom. They could still see a shadow, a bit of tumor residue. Dr. Finn led the discussion among the team, and there was agreement that, while they had the positioning nailed, he would get all of it. A collective deep breath, and Dr. Finn went back in.

The shadow took longer. I was squeezing. I was moving. I was okay. Dr. Finn asked for a different instrument. A man's voice apologized—the suite is so new, it's not completely outfitted—he came back with something else. Dr. Finn said, "This'll work." And it did: Dr. Finn got the shadow. There was the pause again, we were waiting, and this time the images came up clean.

Ding dong, the tumor's gone!

"Suzy, it looks great. We got it all." *See—he doesn't need anybody else's healing statements!* "We'll do a frozen biopsy here, have some preliminary results in the morning—it doesn't look like anything, but I'll have a full pathology report, be able to say for sure in a week." And he left.

The hard part was done. The rest was cake. The first part backwards. Now I wanted my music; I didn't need to hear what they were saying anymore. Two hours to close me up (three CDs), and I was—we were—all home free.

1. SENTENCE DEPARTS BRAIN:

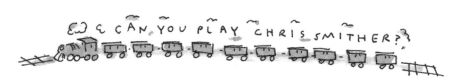

2. EN ROUTE...

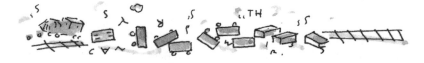

3 . ARRIVES MOUTH :

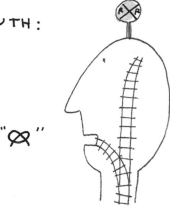

"∞"

I had the whole team's attention. I tried again. This time, the words fell out of the cars before the train left the station.

NOW DEPARTING ON

TRACK 1   HELP.

TRACK 2   CHRIS SMITHER.

TRACK 3   OH MY GOD. OH MY GOD.

TRACK 4   GET DR. FINN. GET

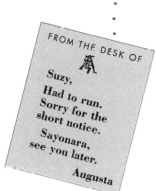

FROM THE DESK OF

Suzy,
Had to run.
Sorry for the
short notice.
Sayonara,
see you later.

Augusta

"Help," I managed.

"It's her speech," someone said, and someone else went to get Dr. Finn.

"Suzy"—Dr. Finn was back—"are you having trouble speaking?"

My tongue was stuck to the top of my mouth. "Nnnnyeah." *Jesusohgod.*

Dr. Finn talked to the team. "She was fine when I left. The images are clear. I am betting it's the swelling, which means it may get worse before it gets better, but it should disappear within twenty-four hours."

Fine? How do you know I was fine? My right side was fine, but no one ever asked me to say anything except okay okay okay. I can say—wait, if I can say okay, I can say—"CD."

"She wants her CDs, her music," somebody interpreted.

"Sssss." *No.* "Cks." *Chris Smither.*

"I can't understand her." *Steve's talking.* Dr. Finn was gone again. "We don't need her for this part—can't we just put her out?"

No. No. NO. I don't want to be put out. I shut up. I wanted to be awake.

After I quieted down, they forgot I was there. Talk turned to TGIF. *F as in the Friday before the Fourth.* "Who's going to Dr. Finn's barbecue? . . . Is it any good? . . . I heard he grills. . . . Where is it?"

I tried mouthing the address. *I don't want to forget any of this.*

"There's a ton of food upstairs. . . ." *Must be getting close to lunchtime.* Talk dropped off. The images were slowing things down. Now the intercom was insisting on another set; blood had pooled in the surgical cavity.

Steve let all but one of the residents go upstairs. I wondered how he picked who got to stay—on the basis of skill or comfort? Either way, he sounded much more relaxed. They put the piece of my skull back on with miniature Erector Set–style plates. Then they sutured the skin, tied off the last stitch, and their work was done.

I was wheeled out of the room, the drapes were lifted off—and they were gone. No good-bye, good luck, no sign of my team anywhere. I was back in Angela's hands. There were murmurs from the staff—accolades: "She looks wonderful. . . . Brain surgery? You'd never know. . . . Look at her color. . . . How do you feel? . . . Why is she crying?"

Put the sheets back over my head. I don't want anybody to see me this way.

"The swelling has affected her speech," Angela explained. "Temporarily."

No one ever said anything like this could happen. . . .

"Well, she *looks* great."

"She'll be fine," Angela said, and rolled me away. The double doors shut on their voices, then the elevator doors.

The FAMILY REUNION

The elevator opened up on the ninth floor. Neuro-ICU. Angela wheeled me to my room and said good-bye.

My room was dark, the only source of light a fluorescent tube on the wall above my head. The venetian blinds over the window to my left sealed off the outside world.

The ICU nurse announced, "Your family members are on their way up to see you. Shall I send your mother in first?"

I need to stop crying before I see my mother—Send in, god, what is her name? I couldn't think of her name. I could only say no. "No. No. No—"

The nurse came back with a list of names and began to read them off: "Karen Simpson." *That's it!* I nodded, and she left again.

Karen was a silhouette in the doorway. She kissed me on the cheek and searched for a place to rest her hand on my body. I had an oxygen tube up my nose, an IV drip in my left arm, another in my right clavicle, the IV backup in my right hand, and a cap on my right index finger, monitoring the oxygen level in my blood. She held on to the rail on my bed.

"Suz." Away from the door, she looked gray. Her eyes welled up. "I just didn't know if I'd ever see you again." She touched my Pebbles ponytail. "You look so little."

She was shifting from side to side, more like swaying. She tightened her grip on my bed rail, and the ICU nurse looked up. "Everything okay?"

"Actually," Karen answered, "I'm feeling a little dizzy."

"Let's sit you down." The nurse lowered the rail, and I made room on my bed. She rubbed Karen's back. "Feeling better?"

Karen shook her head.

"Drop your head, and take a few deep breaths." Karen put her head between her knees. "Let's try this." The ICU nurse took the tube out of my nose and gave it to Karen.

Karen revived. She looked at me, eyebrows raised, wagging her finger. "Don't you start with me—" The three of us couldn't help laughing.

"Everyone is waiting for the report," Karen said. "I'll tell them you look great"—she counted one on her thumb—"your right side is fine." (Two.)

I nodded. "Un my speech?"

"You're having some difficulties with your speech due to swelling"—she looked over at the nurse for confirmation—"but that should clear up in twenty-four hours."

"Unh the mass."

"Looks benign."

Don't leave me. Karen kissed me good-bye. "I'll be back!"

Meredith and my mother came in next. From the looks of them, they, too, had been afraid they might never see me again.

I tried to talk. The speech originated somewhere in the back of my throat. I had to drop my tongue from my palate (where it was otherwise lodged) to let it past. Whatever made its way over my tongue tripped out of my mouth, which by then felt crooked and stiff on account of the swelling. The end product was unintelligible.

COPING STRATEGY #1: *Hmming (Hmm+ ?, Mm!)*	
PRO	CON
comfortable, easy, surprisingly versatile, not noticeable	limiting

I also tried rehearsing a complete sentence in advance. The final delivery so surprised, hence frightened, me, I started crying all over again, which frightened Meredith. She rubbed my left hand and said, "Suz, you don't have to talk now."

COPING STRATEGY #2: *Rehearsing*	
PRO potentially less limiting	CON laborious, unspontaneous, noticeably unsuccessful

My mother added, "She's being such a perfectionist."

COPING STRATEGY #3: *Not talking*	
PRO less noticeable	CON very limiting, slightly frustrating

Meredith and my mother carried on the conversation without me for a few minutes, and then they left. My sister Robin and Bruce took their places. By then, a schedule for the rest of the night had been worked out.

SEAT TIME	
to 12 A.M.	Bruce
12 A.M. – 4 A.M.	Robin
4 A.M. – 6 A.M.	Meredith
6 A.M.	Karen

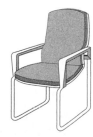

A new private nurse, more like a baby-sitter, arrived every four or six hours with a bag of belongings and a cardigan and disappeared into the corner. She didn't even have to get up to take my blood pressure.

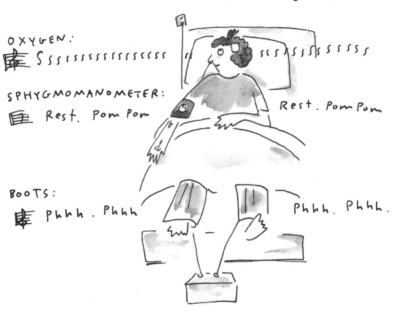

The floor nurse stopped by once or twice an hour to give me pills and administer the reflex and squeeze tests. The private nurse reminded me each time to ask for painkillers *before* the pain got bad. I wasn't feeling any pain— nothing like a migraine. Not the slightest headache. No nausea. Nothing. I rolled over on my side, expecting my hip to object—still nothing.

Except for my speech, I was in very good shape. All my vitals were stable. They took me off the oxygen —ahead of schedule.

My private nurse suggested again that I rest, but I planned to stay up

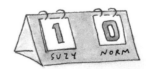

Suzy vs. The Norms

and go to bed at a normal hour. (It always worked for jet lag.) Bruce was sitting in the chair right by my pillow.

He put his left hand under my right. I was feeling tired, but it was hard to fall asleep with all the light in the hall: when I closed my eyes, the insides of my eyelids kept flashing—LIGHT dark (when someone passed by) LIGHT dark LIGHT. After an unusually long darkness, I opened my eyes.

My dad filled the doorway. I'd given up on seeing him. Lightning had struck a control tower in New Hampshire, and they had grounded his flight. "You look wonderful. . . . Doesn't she?" Bruce nodded and got up to give my dad the chair. He just stood beside the bed for a second, looking, until he bent over to kiss me. "I was sitting on that plane—I couldn't call anybody. . . . I'll tell you"—he shook his head—"you are a sight for sore eyes, Suetta." He sat and told me stories about his day on the runway, and I fell fast asleep.

When I awoke, it took a minute to get my bearings. Robin was in the chair. There was a new floor nurse, Night Nurse. *I'm in the hospital.* My private nurse piped up—painkillers. This time I took them. I was beginning to feel the incision. Night Nurse had me retake his neuro tests; he was worried about my *left* side. I must have been overcompensating; he was satisfied the second time.

"Can you tell me your address?"

Your address is not one of those things you have to think about, so I was thinking *Why are you asking me that?* in the same instant I was opening my mouth. Then, nothing came out.

Nothing garbled. Nothing at all.

I am wide awake now. It's all come back to me.

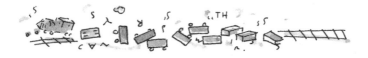

I know my address. How can you know something and not be able to say it? What else can't I say? I can see my house with the number on it. Calm down. If you calm down, it will come back to you.

"Tell me where you are now."

"Hoshpl." *Oh, my god. My mouth is useless. First I have to think of what to say; then I have to tell my mouth how to say it.*

"Do you know the name of the hospital?"

I do. Did. Shit. Wait . . . The train pulled out before the words got on board.

I looked at Robin. She put her hand on my arm.

"Last one: Who's the president?"

I know this. Christ, I worked for him for a year. "I know." *Please give me a second. I can see it; I can say it.* "Clin-ton."

It wasn't much of a victory, but it got him to leave. "I'll be in to check on you again. You should try to get some rest."

I didn't want to rest. I wanted to ace the next check. I asked Robin to go over the questions with me. She'd say the answer, and I'd repeat it back to her. After I had them all down, we talked about other things, waiting for Night Nurse to come back again. Sometimes I would get a whole sentence out. Sometimes a half and Robin filled in the rest. Sometimes I just couldn't give her enough to go on, and it turned into a guessing game, which usually ended with, "It's okay, Suz," and then silence.

```
+-------------------------------+
|      Exam/Assessment          |
+-------------------------------+
| Neuro: -a, 0 x 3              |
|        -expressive aphasia     |
|        no drift                |
|        full strength I all 4 ext.|
|                               |
+-------------------------------+
```

Night Nurse did the squeeze tests first again. *My address is two nine nine South. The president is—Bill, William . . .* I was ready for the next part.

"Tell me what you do."

You never said THAT was going to be on the test!

What I do is . . . I am a _____. What I do is . . . "I do books." I started crying. "Oh, god, Rob."

Night Nurse was concerned. "Okay, where are you?"

Why does it have to be such a goddamn long name? I shook my head.

Robin looked back at Night Nurse. "It's getting worse."

"I'm going to keep checking." One last question: "Who's your doctor?"

"Finn."

Night Nurse left us alone again. "Rob, what *do* I do?" The question scared her, as if now I'd forgotten that, too. "Just how you say—?" I could not remember the words.

"You're an author and an artist."

"Other word? Longer."

"You're an author-illustrator."

That's it. That's what I say. I mimicked the words. *Arthur. Arthau. Arthur is close enough. Arthur-ill.* My tongue quit. *Arthur-Ill-strate. Arthur-Artist.*

See if I can say the book title: All I Can Know I Learn from My Cat.

My speech is getting worse. Not better.

I was afraid to go to sleep.

And wake up with no words at all.

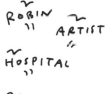

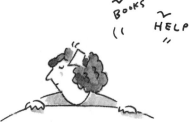

One of the residents made her rounds. She was friendly, close to my age. She administered the neuro tests gently, not tentatively, and quietly checked the chart at the foot of my bed. "Everything looks good!" She smiled and turned to go.

Do not leave me! HELP! I need medical attention! I am losing my words— "Umn. My shpeech?"

"Did Dr. Finn explain about the swelling?"

"He—said—it would get—better."

"It's getting worse," Robin interjected. "Did you talk to the night nurse? I think he's also worried."

"I—NEED—my words—'m scared." I could see we were getting through to her.

"If it gets much worse, we'll send you down for a CAT scan, just to make sure there's nothing else going on. The nurse can page me. I'm on call. I'll let him know."

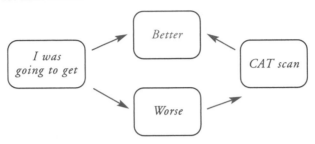

I didn't care if they had to go back in—rip out the stitches, unscrew the plates—not if it would fix my speech. Better before everything started to grow back together. And it'd have to be easier, at least quicker than the first time.

It was a while before Night Nurse came back. He had a new line of questioning. "What's this?" He held up the stuffed dog that Bruce had given me.

I wanted to say *dog,* but *dog* was gone. I hunted around for it; then I settled for *Mister.*

"Mister's her dog," Robin explained. Night Nurse looked less worried. "What's this?"

Pen. I could see it. *P-E-N.* Poof! Gone. "I know."

"That's all right." He set it down. "I know you know."

I liked Night Nurse. "Wait, do it again." He held up the pen. I took it from him and scrawled big capital letters on a scrap of paper before they disappeared. I showed him. "There."

"What does it say?"

Serious? We all know what it says. I read the letters silently. So silently, it was eerie. I could have heard a pin drop in my head. There was no little voice reading out loud in there, queuing up the words, telling me what to say. I was going to have to sound it out. *I was going to have to learn to read out loud all over again, like a six- or five-, four- or three-year-old, or however old they are when they start to read out loud now.*

"I think we're going to send you down for a CAT scan before it gets too busy down there," Night Nurse said. "I'll page the doctor to get you scheduled."

When we were alone again, I asked, "Rob, will I be okay?"

"Suz, I *think* you're going to be okay."

Everyone in our family is so earnest! "I mean like *this*. IF THIS IS ME—IT—ALL—HOW I AM, will THAT be okay?" My frustration had been hardwired to my volume control. I'd made her cry. "Sorry."

Around 4 A.M., Meredith took Robin's place. Dad was sleeping in the air-conditioned room at her place; otherwise, she said, it was too hot to sleep. Her dogs had been up all night, pacing. The hospital, on the other hand, was freezing. She climbed into bed next to me, and it could have been thirty years ago, the two of us in a twin bed, until my parents came upstairs and made us go back to our own beds.

We were awakened by Night Nurse, making his last appearance. I watched him open the blinds a little, letting in first light. I was grateful, full of gratitude I couldn't express. Night Nurse had been how I'd imagined the anesthesiologist would be: there, all through the night.

The final round of squeeze tests was silent; he led and I followed. And then, the final questions: "What day is today?"

I didn't want to cry, not during our last visit. I pointed to the wall.

He smiled and nodded as he tore off the page. Points for cleverness. July 3, Saturday. "I know you know. One more, what time is it?"

"After six—before seven." He wrote 6:25 on his clipboard and held it out. I could *read* the numbers—I could read the hands on the clock, for that matter. . . . I counted up to six. Up to two. Up to five. "Six—two—five." There was something missing, something else to it. . . . *I can't tell time.*

"Someone will be in to take you down for your CAT scan this morning." He gave his clipboard a tug, and I let go.

Meredith asked what time the Au Bon Pain opened downstairs. "Can I? . . . Coffee?" I asked. My ice-chip-and-water diet was not officially over until hospital breakfast was served.

"I don't see why not." It made him smile, getting to say something that made me happy.

Meredith came back with a cup for each of us. I closed my eyes and disappeared in the steam—vaporized—having coffee in Paris, Cambridge, anywhere else, but—"Suzy Becker?" I put my cup on the tray, and the attendant wheeled me, bed and all, to radiology. I wasn't afraid. I wasn't hopeful. Or maybe I was both, and they canceled each other out. I just wanted to get better. Whatever it took to get better.

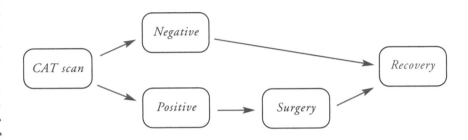

The CAT scan was negative. There was no abnormality in the surgical cavity. No reason to go back in. No explanation, then, for my deterioration. *But Dr. Finn would know—would have to know—what it was and when it would go away. He would have some explanation why. Besides, it hasn't even been twenty-four hours.*

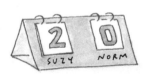

As soon as I got back the day nurse removed my catheter. "We're going to get you out of here, move you up to the tenth floor this morning," she said with a smile.

Morning stretched into afternoon. No one said anything as Karen, Bruce, and the rest of my family (six over one-person limit) crowded in. We passed the time modeling the headband-hats a friend had made for me.

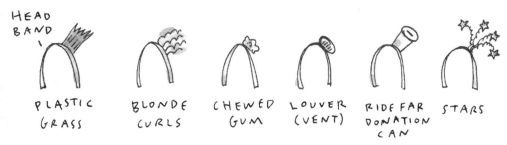

HEAD BAND

PLASTIC GRASS   BLONDE CURLS   CHEWED GUM   LOUVER (VENT)   RIDE FAR DONATION CAN   STARS

The day nurse commandeered a wheelchair at 2 P.M. We packed up the hats, figuring the move was at hand. *Forget my speech, I can't wait to watch Wimbledon on the TV in my new room.* When 3:30 (the end of her shift) rolled around and she still hadn't located an aide, the nurse decided she would wheel me up to the tenth floor herself.

My new room, 10-D, was a double—and I was the first one in it. I picked the side with the bed by the window (and the shared bathroom). Karen helped me change into the button-front pajama top my mother had lent me, a pair of flannel boxers, and the black hat we'd picked out after the mention of the treatment plan. (It looked good with or without hair.) I was ready to receive visitors again.

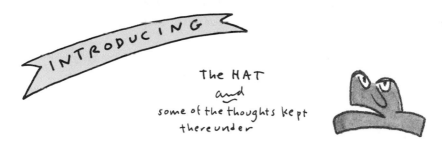

INTRODUCING

The HAT
and
some of the thoughts kept
thereunder

It was a family reunion of sorts. (The last time my mother and father had been in the same place at the same time was during Robin's jewelry show opening, four summers before.) Karen sat to my immediate left. Meredith; her fiancé, Jonathan; Robin; and my mother filled out the left flank, along the radiator. My dad sat in a chair on my right, near the foot of the bed.

Before she had left, the ninth-floor nurse had encouraged me to try sitting up in the chair for short periods of time. Karen and I traded places, so Karen was lying on my bed when the tenth-floor nurse walked in. She nodded at Karen and went directly into the bathroom. While she was in the bathroom, Karen and I quietly switched back.

When the nurse emerged from the bathroom, she explained how she would be monitoring my—she glanced at Karen, then at me—eliminations. After that, we saw her only at pill time. She'd set the condiment cup and a glass of water on the tray, scarcely looking at who was in the bed.

At one point, she admonished us to keep it down, and she nudged my father's chair (with my father in it) closer to the bed for emphasis. My roommate had arrived. I caught a glimpse of her—a little older than me, thin brown hair, with a bandage on the back of her head—before the nurse whisked the curtain shut behind my father.

The divider made for a hemmed-in feeling on our side of the room. It was no longer possible to see the hallway, to watch for Dr. Finn.

Conversation starters were thrown out, like streamers, not aimed at anyone in particular. They hung in the air for a few seconds, then died. That was when my mother said she slept the whole night through for the first time since Paris. After leaving the hospital, she had phoned three of her closest friends, skipped dinner, and gone straight to bed. Once she'd said that, I noticed she looked rested. And dressed up. She had dressed up for the hospital and my father.

Now that I had survived the surgery, everyone else was beginning to break down. There were these time bombs, getting ready to go off:

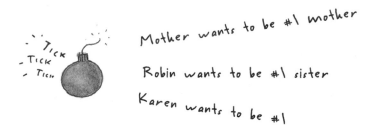

Mother wants to be #1 mother

Robin wants to be #1 sister

Karen wants to be #1

Dr. Finn's visit broke through the haze of the late afternoon. He circled the bed, introducing himself to everyone with a handshake. My dad, several inches taller than Dr. Finn, rested his left hand on Dr. Finn's upper right arm, almost an embrace—

 I know it's a Saturday, but you can all QUIT being so impressed and indebted and help me get my words back!

Dr. Finn said, "The surgery went extremely well. We got all of the tissue, and our frozen sample was negative—that's to say not cancerous."

Everybody looked relieved, and I guess I was, too, even though the fear of cancer had seemed so remote.

"We won't have the full lab report for several days. . . ." He turned to me. "How are you feeling?"

"Ng." Tongue, stuck again, on the roof of my mouth. "Ngood. Except my speech." I pointed at my mouth in lieu of another sentence.

"You *look* good. I like the hat.
And you *sound* pretty good to me. What's giving
you the trouble?"

Harrumph.

"Numbers—time—address."

Robin added, "She can't say what she does. Sorry, Suz, is this? Should I? . . . She couldn't identify lots of things, like a pen. It got worse through the night, although, it was kind of funny, she could always say *your* name."

Dr. Finn smiled and put his hands in his white coat pockets. "A thousand neurosurgeons could not have predicted this result—of course, we all knew Suzy's brain was a little unusual but—"

Everybody laughed.

Hartyharharhar.

Recovery Clock

"We expect this will go away."

"You said tw-th. Hou—" I couldn't get the numbers out.

Robin said them for me: "Twenty-four hours."

"Let's give it another twenty-four, see how you're doing tomorrow."

48 hours

"The barbecue at your house? . . . Chethster Square?" His home address surprised him. "I heard." *Everything, I mean.* "You grill?"

He laughed and shook his head. "You're going to be fine."

I turned the TV on. My mother went out to have a cigarette. When she came back, Robin stood up. She was about to say something difficult. "Mother, we should go soon. I have to go to Suzy's. Mister's been in his crate all this time." Her chin quivered; the hard part was coming. "I'm not answering your phone." She looked at me. "I'll let the machine . . . they're going to ask me how you're doing, and I can't lie."

Karen was next to me, on the bed. "You don't have to lie."

My father seconded, "No one's asking you to lie."

Robin's expression was worsening by the minute; she was

falling down before she even got to the job. In the rush to get out of my mouth, my words all balled up.

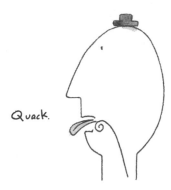

Quack.

Try again, s l o w l y. "Okay. Take messages."

My mother whispered to Robin, "She doesn't sound like herself."

"I heard!" I started to cry.

"She got upset when I said she sounded fine—I just can't say the right thing." My mother was crying, too. She turned and walked out of the room.

Robin followed her. My father tsked, shaking his head sadly. Meredith and Jonathan instantly agreed it was time for dinner and took my father with them, promising to bring back ice cream.

Karen and I were alone, and I was still crying. *This* is *myself. This* is *myself.* Karen held me.

When Bruce came back, he took Karen out for dinner, and I was alone. *For the first time since*—(I couldn't remember when)—*I am all by myself.*

I kept the TV off. And the lights off. I watched the twilight infuse the sky. Not talking. Not listening. Not yet afraid of the nothingness in my head. Resting.

My roommate was resting, too. The room was quiet, just the sound of inflating boots. Her side of the room had been quiet—no visitors, no phone calls—all day. Then I heard her start to make a noise. She was about to throw up. I rang for the nurse, and I pointed at the curtain.

She came back to check on me when she was through with my room-mate. *Can I walk can I walk can I walk.* "Can I walk?"

"You'll need one of us to assist you, and we're short-staffed tonight. I'll see if I can make it back." She never did.

"You're so lucky you feel like getting up and walking around." My roommate was talking to me; I sat up to see if I could see her. "I feel so nauseous all the time."

I wanted to say, "You're so lucky you can say *nauseous*," but I couldn't begin to string the words together. "Mm."

I'm a disappointment as a roommate. To myself. After all the TV shows, all the books I'd read, after all the years I'd had to imagine the kind of patient I would be.

GOOD PATIENTHOOD

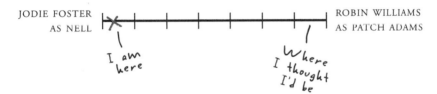

I lay back down.

Eventually, Bruce and Karen came back, and my dad and Meredith dropped off a pint of Ben & Jerry's with two spoons. Bruce and I lay on the bed, eating ice cream, channel surfing, and looking out at the city.

"Pretty," Bruce said, about the view.

"Where is it?" I asked. He shrugged. It didn't matter; it was pretty.

There were long stretches of silence between us. The kind you can have when you talk every day. There's no rush, no backlog of things left unsaid.

When I was tired, I rolled away from the window and slept. No private nurses. No neurological testing every hour on the tenth floor. The minimum maintenance plan.

I couldn't get back to sleep after my middle-of-the-night pill delivery. The TV was still on, but that wasn't keeping me up—I'd had too much rest. "Bruce, you awake?"

"Haven't slept." The tenth floor was still.

"You get a nurse, I walk?"

COPING STRATEGY #4: *Minimum words plan*	
PRO effective	CON caveman-like

He went to see to what he could do. "Someone's coming," he said, and he sat in the chair instead of getting back into bed.

I let the nurse slide off my boots (even though I'd already removed and replaced them once myself when I couldn't wait any longer and Karen had to help me hobble to the bathroom). She put hospital slippers over my surgical hose and set my feet shoulder-width apart onto the floor. Then she held my left arm, inside the elbow, and tugged me off the bed. I straightened, pausing, preparing to walk. Standing, I noted, felt fine.

> You're walking. And you don't always realize it, / but you're always falling. / With each step you fall forward slightly. / And then catch yourself from falling. / Over and over, you're falling. / And then catching yourself from falling.
>
> —LAURIE ANDERSON,
> "WALKING AND FALLING"

I slid the slippers forward, left, right; then took small steps. The foam grabbed the floor reassuringly. I pulled the nurse in tighter to keep from listing to the right. Then I tried compensating, putting more weight on my left slipper. After a couple more steps, the nurse let go. "I'm going to let your husband (I could feel Karen cringing) take it from here." Bruce caught my elbow, and we proceeded to circle the hallways surrounding the nurses' station.

The rooms were dark; I would have had to strain to look in. As bad as I felt, I sensed I was better off than most. But I did not want to *know;* I did not want to *see.* Their faces would get in the way when I went to put my needs first.

Bruce helped me put my boots back on, and I lay back in bed. Reality *(walking is a milestone for an eighteen-month-old)* is suspended in the hospital; I fell asleep feeling satisfied.

Hospital
Milestone

FIREWORKS

I'd forgotten what day it was until I saw Karen in her stars-and-stripes shirt and matching flip-flops. She had a box full of stuff: a big flag, which Bruce helped her hang by the window, a red plastic ball, and a breakfast-at-Wimbledon picnic. Karen loves the Fourth of July more than anybody I've ever known—the fireworks and the fact it's not a family holiday. She doesn't have any siblings, and her parents are both dead.

I took off my boots and put on my slippers. We decided to walk Bruce out and get some coffee and *The New York Times*. An almost normal Sunday.

My roommate was sitting up, alone, finishing the hospital-issue breakfast when we got back to the room. We exchanged "Mornings" as Karen unrolled our cloth place mats and poured us real orange juice into plastic goblets. We had almond croissants on picnic plates. I ate the hospital bran muffin when it showed up, although the Starbuck's from downstairs had already created the stirrings of success.

The nurse came by to check. "Any bowel—?" I nodded. Meredith, Jonathan, and my dad were in the doorway.

Getting out of the Hospital Checklist

✓ Get catheter out
✓ Get out of ICU
✓ Get off IVs
✓ Eat
✓ Walk
(Poop)

They had stopped at a florist's on their way in. My dad handed me a plant. It was familiar, but I couldn't recall the name. I read the tag several times and tried to sound it out silently.

The newspaper was passed around. I avoided picking it up. When my mother arrived at a little past noon with a box of pastries, I still had not laid eyes on a single section. *Give it another twenty-four hours.*

How 'bout I call you "plant"?!

My name is Hibiscus rosa sinensis but you can call me "Hibiscus"

NOT EDIBLE

My dad was embarking on the crossword. He read out the first clue, and I was shocked. It was completely out of character. My dad's idea of sharing the puzzle has always been making and distributing photocopies before he uncaps his pen and we all work in silence.

Meredith, Jonathan, and my mother didn't even look up. Karen was resting in bed beside me. My dad repeated the clue. Karen sat up, and I stopped watching TV.

"How many letters?" Karen asked.

I took the two pieces of information we were given, and I set them out, waiting for my brain to swoop down, snap them up, and spit out an answer, like always.

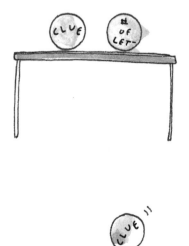

I waited half a minute.

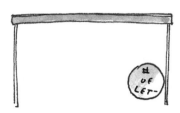

I asked for the clue a third time. This time I tried to recall what it was I wanted my brain to do with the information: *Search,* I prompted my brain. *Sort by number of letters.* My brain couldn't search.

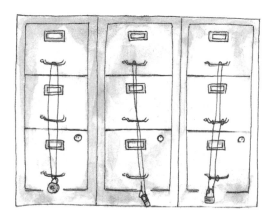

It offered up a weak guess and left me to count the letters on my fingers. "Dad, I can't."

He gave me a different clue.

"Stop. I can't. I can't think of the word. AND how many letters." My first cry of the day. "I can't do puzzles." I turned my head into Karen's shoulder. I wanted to disappear inside my hat. Everyone was quiet.

My dad continued to read an occasional clue, always directed at somebody other than me. *Water torture.* I concentrated on the ceiling; my tolerance threshold was creaking when Karen nudged me. "Wanna go for a walk?"

We did the nurses' station circuit and got back in bed. Same scene, ten minutes later. Karen closed her eyes. I was thinking about closing my eyes just because it was easier than keeping them open when Robin arrived. She was visibly calmer, having successfully fielded the morning's phone calls, a total of twenty-eight.

My friend Ellen and her husband, Alex, walked in on Robin's heels. Ellen and I were roommates at Brown.

If conversation is like tennis, Ellen returns everything I send over, and sometimes hits it back twice as fast. And if I were the emperor, she'd tell me I had no clothes.

IMPENETRABLE
FORCE FIELD

"How are you?"

I pulled my hat down. "Good."

"Nice hat." Ellen smiled.

I smiled back, hoping someone else would take up the conversational slack. Meredith introduced Jonathan, and it turns out they lived just a few blocks apart—the conversation was going; I could rest.

After Ellen and Alex left, it was just the family again. Wimbledon was over. Karen was asleep. My mother went out for a cigarette, and Meredith went to keep her company. No sign of Dr. Finn. *I don't know if I can take another day in the hospital.* "Want to walk?" I asked Robin. "To see the fireworks. Where to see the fireworks." We left my dad with Jonathan and Karen, who was still sleeping.

As we neared the nurses' station, I dropped behind Robin. (Historically, I'd been the talker in these situations.) "We were going to try to find a place to watch the fireworks," she half announced, half asked the nurse on duty.

"Top floor." Seemed obvious.

"Is there a roof?" Robin followed up. *There's a roof on* ER. . . .

"No. Ask once you're up there." Dismissed.

We'd only taken a few steps off the elevator when we were approached. "May I help you?" There was no mistaking me for a visitor.

Robin started to explain.

"There are critically ill cardiac patients on this floor. "

"It's just that one of the nurses on the tenth floor—"

"You'll have to find an empty room."

"Can you tell us which *side* would be better—?"

"I'm not a night nurse. I've never seen the fireworks. I couldn't tell you anything."

No one else bothered us as we traipsed around the halls, peering out window after window. Finally we found an empty room with a view of the river. Robin memorized the location, and we headed back down to the tenth floor. Meredith and my mother were sitting on a bench right outside the elevator; the cigarette break had segued into a candy bar break.

"Mommy hasn't eaten a meal since I've been here," Robin told me on our way back to the room. "She's living off candy bars."

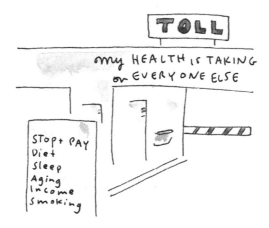

My dad was talking to Jonathan; Karen appeared to be sleeping. "I don't know of any friend who would spend two nights in a hospital—Bruce has been that kind of friend since—when did you meet Bruce, Suetta?"

Second Ride FAR. 1990. 1999 minus 1990. "Ten"—*Christ, that's so annoying*—"nine years."

I reached over Karen for my boots, and her eyes popped open. "Can I talk to you for a minute? Outside?" I dropped the boots.

"I can't take it anymore. I can't do this. I can't. I can't. I am your lover, your partner. What do they think I am doing here? I've hardly left the hospital. I haven't eaten. I haven't taken care of myself. I have had *no* time for myself; I'm behind in everything . . . and I have to sit there, sit there and listen to how wonderful Bruce is— Why don't you goddamn marry him?" Her head ended up in her hands, her elbows on her knees. I could barely get my arms around her.

"Sweetie . . ." She looked up, still sobbing. It was the first time I'd seen her look all fifty-one years. "Please."

"Your father hates me." *He doesn't. He's loved you from the first time, the first Thanksgiving.* Karen helped him buy a camera. "I am lying there, resting, and he knows—*he knows*—and he says to Jonathan how thankful he is you have Bruce. How *Bruce* is always there for you. I have to get out of here."

Me, too. I have struggled (and failed) to help you see or feel you are the most important person in my life in the eleven months up until now, and now, now I can only say, "Dad loves you. Don't go—like this—*I* love you."

The elevator doors opened, and it was Bruce, wearing red, white, and blue Converse sneakers and a pair of oversize sunglasses. After one look at us, he removed them and went ahead to the room. "I'm going to see if I can find someone to go to the fireworks with me. I'm sorry, Suz—" the storm had passed—"I can't stay here, I need to—"

"It's okay—Patty?"

"I was going to try her first. Please don't say anything about this. Don't say anything to your father."

"I won't." She came back to the room, and I watched her gather up her things.

She kissed my father good-bye. My dad stood. "You'll have to come to Philadelphia; there are a couple of really great little places we would love to take you—as soon as the patient—"

"We're going to need a vacation." Karen smiled. She kissed me good-bye. "You rest." She pointed to the bed.

I walked her to the elevator, then hesitated before climbing back into bed. I stood with my back to the radiator, facing my father, waiting until I had everyone's attention.

"Um. About Karen. Is my partner." *Shit.* I was already crying. "Did all this. You need to love her. Nn, show her."

Meredith put her arm around me. My mother eyed Robin nervously. My dad tsked.

I got in bed and put my boots back on. An orderly arrived with my dinner, saw Bruce in his outfit sitting below the flag, and said, "Y'all having a party on this side?" No one answered.

My dad was standing. I moved my dinner away and got up to hug him good-bye. "I'm glad I was here. I don't know that I was too much of a help, but—" He touched my hair gingerly and glanced at my mother. "Good-bye, Lois."

My mother nodded from her chair. Robin met him at the corner of the bed and hugged him good-bye.

He stopped at the edge of the curtain and looked back at me, "I'll call you tomorrow, Suette."

My mother left shortly after my dad. Robin went to feed her dog.

My roommate passed by on her way to the bathroom. I tried not to look at the dressing on the back of her head. *Bloody.* She looked back. "You're up," I said. *Who's luckier now?*

Bruce brought a sandwich back. We watched TV and ate in bed. He crumpled up his sandwich foil, shot, and missed the wastebasket. When he got up to dunk the foil, he grabbed the red ball. "Two square?"

The nurse checked her watch as we walked past the station. "Not time for the fireworks, already, is it?" She hadn't noticed the ball. "Let me give you your blood thinner while you're here." She lifted my pajama top; my stomach was mottled from two days' worth of injections. "Wouldn't hurt if you had a little more fat around your middle," she joked, and stuck me. I pinched the spot to dull the burn, helping the next bruise along. She sat back down.

Bruce and I set up our two-square court out of view, back by the freight elevator.

TWO-SQUARE COURT

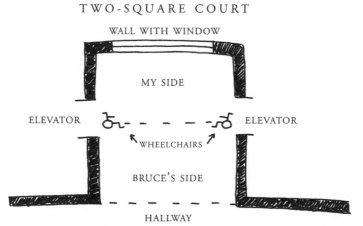

An automatic time-out was called when the elevator doors opened and two white coats emerged, engrossed in conversation. They pushed the half-court wheelchair out of their way and continued down the hall. Play resumed. I was up by a couple of points (and doing better with my numbers, keeping score), having fun, you could almost say—when Bruce sent a ball to the back right corner. I lunged for it. *Shit.* I felt a surge in my head. GAME OVER! *Stupid! What if you've ruptured something? Please, don't make it worse. I promise to be more careful.* I took Bruce's arm and retreated to my bed.

ICP
ALERT!

There was no sign of Robin when it was time for the fireworks. The elevator was packed with patients—ambulatory and wheelchair —and unusually empty of medical personnel. Bruce and I were last in, first out. We headed down the hall to claim our room. The rest of the group looked after us, bobbed in unison, then headed in the opposite direction.

We found an empty room, not exactly where I'd remembered it, and sat on the bed, staring out toward the water. There was no TV hookup, no simulcast, so it was hard to gauge the actual start time. After ten minutes of nothing, we bailed and went to find the rest of the group. A nurse was herding them out of one room and into another; Robin was with them.

The new room was all dark, except for the monitors. The patients' hearts beat steadily, one faster than the other's. They appeared to be sleeping very deeply. Or in comas.

The nine or ten of us filed in and silently arranged ourselves between the one bed and the window. Wheelchairs and short people in front, wheelchair pushers in next, and the rest, in back, practically on the bed. I knelt beside a woman in a wheelchair. She poked me and said in a raspy whisper, "We oughtta turn the TV on."

I gave a noncommittal "hm." I didn't agree with her, but I didn't want to disagree or ignore her altogether, causing her to raise her voice, which would have resulted in the same outcome (waking up our hosts) as turning on the TV.

She leaned her head back and said upside down, loudly, "Phil, turn on the TV. It's gonna take more than TV to wake these people up." *Living proof.* "Half the show is the music. More than half." She was talking to herself now. Phil said nothing. "Phil, I've had enough of this, take me back to the room."

Everyone moved so they could get out. It was silent again. She was right; it wasn't much of a show. The fireworks were the size of dandelion heads. Our elevator-mates left one or two at a time until it was just Robin, Bruce, and me. I'd looked forward to it too much to leave before it ended. Somewhere, over on the other side of the river, Karen was watching.

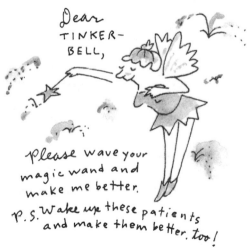

After Bruce and Robin left, I picked up the phone to call Karen—the 11 P.M. check-in. There was no dial tone. I pushed *8* to get out. No luck. I tried *9*. Nothing. I hung up the phone and felt a cry coming on. *I don't want to be all alone, not yet. I'm not even tired.*

Bruce walked back in; he'd forgotten the big sunglasses. "Need—for work?" It was an attempt at a joke, but more of a cover-up for my crying.

"Want some help?" He picked up the phone.

"No tone."

He looked up at the bulletin board. "Did you try that?" There was a seven-digit access number posted. Big block numbers: 791-5786. The second I looked away from the board and down at the receiver, the numbers were gone. *Just the first three: 7-9-1. The first two? What does the dash mean?* The push-button tones were loud and disorienting. *I am even worse than I thought.*

Bruce took the receiver. "You calling Karen?"

I nodded.

"Tell me her number again."

Oh, god.

"Six-one-seven—" He paused.

6-1-7, 6-1-7, I repeated to myself.

"I can't."

Bruce called Information and dialed the number. When Karen picked up, he handed me the phone, kissed me on the forehead, and left again. "Hi." After all that trouble, I had nothing to say; nothing to catch up on, and no incentive to think of something to say when I wouldn't be able to say it anyway.

"Sorry, Suz. I'm sorry I lost it. I think I just needed a break."

"I know."

"Did you get to see the fireworks?"

"Mm. It was funny." Too hard to explain. "Did Patty?"

"She came, and we watched from this side of the river. Next year, we'll watch 'em together. . . ."

"I miss you." *I missed the fireworks with you. I miss you now. I miss sleeping with you. I miss—*

"I miss you, too, Suz. You should rest, I'll see you in the morning."

"And?" (That's what *she* always said.)

"I love you."

"Love you, too."

I still wasn't sleepy. The effect of going to bed is lost on someone who's been in bed all day. I listened to the boots, breathing in and out. *Now I lay me down to sleep, I pray the ? my brain to keep.*

WALKING PAPERS

Just after dawn, the night nurse said good-bye and wished me good luck. "They're sending you home. They would have sent you home yesterday if it hadn't been a Sunday *and* a holiday."

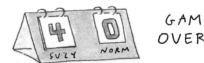

GAME
OVER!!!!

"Will I see Dr. Finn?"
"On a holiday? What am I saying? Dr. Finn's always around. . . ."
I couldn't get back to sleep.

Things I could not *do to pass the time*

Get coffee too early
Shower not allowed
Watch TV only paid thru 7/4
Listen to music too early
Talk on the phone too early + too hard
Read impossible
Write? haven't tried

I opened my mouth in a yawn to stretch my jaw and felt a ping around the incision. My face was getting stiffer by the day, from the swelling, I supposed, but I still had no real pain to complain about.

I decided to pack . . . leaving the boots on. The cord stretched from my bed to the wall, where I'd left the box I'd brought. Meredith's birthday presents were sitting, wrapped, on the bottom. *Today's her birthday. Wow, I used to think of everything. . . .* I put them on the tray. I unplugged my CD player and lowered it into the box, along with the CDs; the hats; the good-luck stuffed animals, bracelet, necklaces, and brass heart—the jury was still out on them. I shut the box and looked around the room.

The plants—*no room:* I'd leave them for my roommate. And there was my book bag, with all the work I thought I'd do, sitting on the floor by the radiator. I opened it up and extracted my notebook, sandwiched between the John Irving book and some Ride FAR files. I took my pencil tin out of the zippered pocket and put it on top of the book next to the presents on my tray. *Maybe I'll try writing.*

I climbed back into bed, considered the notebook, and then pushed the tray aside. *After breakfast. With a cup of coffee from downstairs—*

"Becker—" I heard my name in the hall. "—midthirties. Tolerated the surgery extremely well." It was Steve, the resident, the first time I'd seen him since he shaved my head.

I checked the mirror to make sure my hat was on right—when I looked back, I caught the last of his flock fluttering by. "She's reported some difficulties with speech, but she's young. She'll be fine. With an older patient . . ." His voice trailed off.

Excuse me, I'd mistaken you for someone who gave a shit.

I left my boots at the bottom of the bed and went downstairs for coffee. "Coffee with expresso"—*ESSpresso!*—"please."

"The Red Eye?"

I nodded. *Whatever your little name is for it. I'm not up to menu reading today.* I stepped back onto the elevator with my coffee. Two youngish doctors were midconversation.

They weren't discussing a patient. They might have been students—I tried to get a sideways look. Then I looked right at them, my prerogative as a sick person. They looked away.

Information about patients is confidential and should never be discussed in public places. Thank you for respecting our patients' privacy.

And kindly refrain from staring at them.

Back in bed, I put my coffee down and picked up my notebook. There was at least an hour before Karen arrived. I flipped through the pages, gazing at my handwriting. *I'm pretty sure I'll be able to read these thoughts, just, will I ever be able to* think *them again?*

I opened to a clean left-hand page.

July 5, 1999

The first time I *decided* ~~to~~ ~~able~~ to write.
& summoning up the courage.
~~My~~ right hand side is fine, but my speech, writing, reading abilities are screwed up. ~~messed up.~~

Dr. Finr said 1000 neurosurgeons could not have not predict~~ed to~~ the results ~~to~~ maybe something to do with my unusual language bundling.
I don't recognize numbers. Or say my street address. or what I do. I am afraid ~~d~~ to draw.

The 3 most big ~~important~~ important things.
FUCK Noone said any thing

Noone ~~ever~~ ~~too~~ cares.

ALL I NEED TO KNOW ~~FEE~~ I LEARNED FROM MY CAT.

about speech.

handwriting will ~~come~~ back.

I'm an author and illustrator. ~~It eat~~ comes out like a tongue twister. I could cartoonist yesterday. Everybody thinks I'll be fine. So ~~many~~ maybe I will be.

I laid my head back to rest. A thousand neurosurgeons couldn't answer my questions: *Will I be able to write again? Teach again? Will I ever get my life back?*

I wondered if copying sentences out of the newspaper was any easier than making them up. The sports section was within reach.

as a compliment to America's Mia Hamm.
I think this is enough for today.

I snapped the notebook shut, then opened it again.

I'll ~~do~~ fucking ~~this~~ give up my right side
for my speech & reading. Thanks for
~~the~~ asking.

Karen arrived. I shut the notebook again.

"What's wrong, Suz?"

"Writing."

She was thrilled. "Let me see!"

I'd never let her look at my notebook before. "Not now."

As soon as the tenth-floor nurse could locate someone from the ultrasound department (closed, holiday Monday) to confirm there were no blood clots in my legs, I could go home. She'd paged the head of the department but hadn't heard back. She had, however, located a shower chair, and as soon as she could get her hands on it, she would get me showered. (There was no point in asking whether I could shower without the chair when I knew the answer: patient must shower *with* chair before showering without—and I'd be home for my second shower.)

The nurse showed Karen how to change my bandage. My head, according to Karen, wasn't nearly as bloody as my roommate's, and my hair was already starting to grow back. I didn't want to look.

The nurse covered the new bandage so it was waterproof. She eyed my side of the room. "You're all packed up and ready to go, huh?" I nodded. She looked at her watch. "Eight A.M. Let me go page ultrasound again."

A few minutes later, she was back with our shower chair. "I have several other patients I need to take care of. Do you think you—?" She steered the chair toward Karen.

"Of course." Karen wheeled the chair over to the shower, and the nurse shut the door to the room on her way out.

The two of us stepped inside a bathroom that was roughly one and a half times the size of an airplane's. Karen stacked my pajamas behind the open john, then reassessed and chucked them out on the chair by the bed.

She adjusted the water temperature, then pointed at the seat like the Ghost of Christmas Past. I looked hesitatingly at the sagging wet seat, resigned myself, and sat down. Karen pushed the chair forward, and the back legs bucked. I stood so she could manually redirect each wheel toward the shower, then sat back down—stood—sat—stood. We gave up. I leaned on Karen, who was soaked by this point, while she washed my body; then I sat in the chair so she could wash my hair.

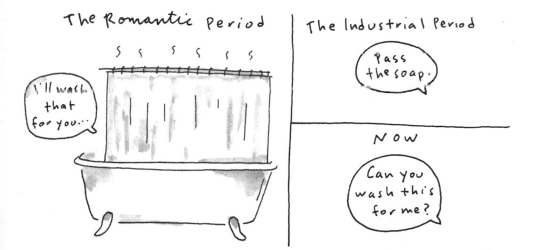

My Cosmetics Bag

Q-tips
deodorant
lotion
toothbrush
toothpaste
floss

The bathroom door, when it was opened at a right angle, made a little dressing area in the back corner of the room. Karen handed me my "cosmetics" bag.

I put my real clothes back on (the ones I'd worn Friday) and patted my hair dry. Karen and my roommate were watching me in the mirror. "Do you want me to comb it out for you?"

Have you ever, once, in all the time we've been together, seen me comb my hair?!

Karen caught me glaring in the mirror. "Suz, I got the blood out, but it's still matted."

All the more reason not to let a comb near it. I put my hat back on and sat on the bed, waiting for my ultrasound.

Meredith and Jonathan stopped by, coffees in hand. They were supposed to be on vacation in Maine, but they had had to cancel when my surgery was postponed. The cottage owner kept their deposit.

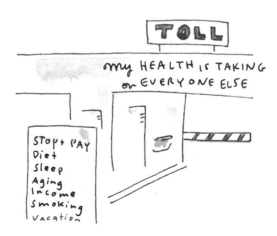

"Here—" I moved the tray toward Meredith. "Happy!" I waved my hand and tried to look happy; I'd never get past the *th* in *birthday*.

Meredith looked down at the presents. "Let's wait until you're better."

If we knew when that would be— I didn't want to have to look at the presents with their little bows every day until then. She took them with her.

The nurse came back to update us; the director of the department herself was on her way in to do my ultrasound. In the meantime, we could get my discharge paperwork out of the way. She sat down on the bed next to me, her pen poised on her clipboard. "Where will you be going?"

I looked at Karen.

Karen answered, "My house." She gave the address.

"Will someone be able to take care of you there?" The nurse was still talking to me, but now she was looking at Karen, too, who nodded. "And"—her pen skipped down the page—"I already showed you how to change the bandage. Once a day, or if it gets wet—it shouldn't get wet— no shampooing around the incision, and call if there are any signs of infection, redness, swelling, tenderness, nausea—it's all written right here—vomiting, any worsening in speech, any weakness, and of course, seizures. Here's your medication schedule." It looked more like a multiplication table; I hoped Karen was following.

The wheelchair had arrived to take me to my ultrasound. (Wheelchair on official business; walking on *unofficial* business only.) "Suzy Becker?"

What's left of her. I let the attendant help me into the chair.

Karen followed us down. The director of the department dismissed the attendant and asked us to wait in the hall; her daughter was with her because she had no day care. "This might take a few extra minutes—it's been a while since I actually had to run one of the machines myself."

The hall felt familiar, which saved it from feeling depressing. No windows, the dim fluorescent overheads, a series of doors—some closed, some open. The rooms themselves were all dark. Patients sat in wheelchairs; one or two lay in hospital beds. Visitors waited in regular chairs to the left and right of the doorways. There was no waiting area, no one to check you in. We were already in the system, quietly waiting our turns.

The director of the department was ready. "Do you need any help getting on the table?"

I went to shake my head—and winced: intracranial pressure. "My head," I explained.

I lay back on the table, and she spread warm gel on my lower leg.

ICP
ALERT!

"I'm checking here for DVTs, deep vein thromboses—clots in the deep veins of your legs. A DVT can travel to the lung and become what's known as a PE, pulmonary embolism." She slid the probe across my skin, through the gel. "You have very beautiful veins," she said. Her voice was soothing; the whole procedure was soothing, in the dark. "Just beautiful."

She turned the monitor toward Karen and me. "Look how clear! You could be an ultrasound model!"

"Do they *pay* people for that?" Karen asked.

"Oh, yes—you know how hard it is to get a good clear picture? This could be a fluke, but—they pay quite a bit for textbooks and overheads." She swiveled the monitor back and prepped my thigh. Now her daughter was interested. The six-year-old studied the monitor; then her mother settled her back down at the desk with more scrap paper.

She picked up where she left off: my groin. I wondered if she could see my ovaries. *I forgot what it was called.* "The other ulterultra—sound?" I said to Karen. Karen explained how I was supposed to have a pelvic ultrasound but we'd postponed it.

"That's farther up." *But maybe since you're in the neighborhood?* "You shouldn't put it off any longer. Your lymph nodes are all full down here."

The sirens were warming up in my head. She squeezed gel on my other calf. Karen asked, "What does that mean, about the lymph nodes?" She tightened her grip on my hand.

"It could mean anything from infection to cancer," she said—like it was "Pass the butter."

Well, why bother going home? Transfer me to the cancer floor, save everybody a trip. It is impossible to think anything is nothing after you've had a stress episode turn into a brain tumor. Tears were running out the corners of my eyes, pooling in my hair. The two of us were silent until she pronounced me "all set."

The attendant wheeled me back up. Karen had me stay in the chair so no one would snag it while she went to find the nurse. "She's printing out your papers."

The nurse came in right behind her, papers in hand. She went over everything one last time. "And, Dr. Finn's office wants you to call once you're settled." Her pen rested on "Follow up appointment," right above

"Return to work" where "Immediately" was filled in. I pointed, attempting a question mark with my eyebrows, but they weren't budging. Swollen. She crossed out "Immediately."

EXCUSE FOR INNER BOSS

Call your doctor if: Temperature higher than 100.5, Draining wound, Any signs of infection, redness, swelling, tenderness, Nausea, Vomiting, Any worsening of speech, weakness in arms or legs, change in vision or mental status any sign of seizure activity

Follow-up appt: Dr. Finn 1 week

Return to work.   ~~Immediately~~ *not till cleared by MD.*

Karen put the plants on my roommate's tray table. She was sleeping, on her back, right on her bloody bandage. *Ow.* I stopped myself. *I can't. I can't worry about you. I am sorry. Good luck. I mean, get well. I hope everything turns out okay.*

I never knew what kind of tumor she had; whether it was her first craniotomy; what her prognosis was—I never got her name—I never learned any of the nurses' names.

GOOD PATIENTHOOD

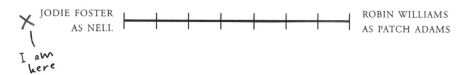

JODIE FOSTER AS NELL ———————————————— ROBIN WILLIAMS AS PATCH ADAMS

X
I am here

Karen put my box on my lap, and away we went. She wheeled me through the lobby and parked me facing out to the pickup area. I caught my reflection in the window and looked away, then looked back harder. *Can people tell this isn't me? Do I look like I belong in a wheelchair?*

When the old silver wagon pulled up, I didn't wait for Karen to come get me. We didn't need to keep up the wheelchair charade while no one was watching—I stood and walked through the revolving door, carrying my box, into a wall of heat.

Karen took the box and started toward the back of the car, then did a 180, realizing she had left me unattended. She hurried around to open the passenger door.

"Thanks," I said.

I'm not an invalid.

She reclined my seat and rolled down my window.

"How do you feel, sweetie?" She was in the driver's seat.

"Not bad." It was probably a hundred degrees, and the car had no air-conditioning. "Hot."

"Let's get you some air-conditioning." She was careful not to say *home*. Her home was not my home. My home was in Bolton.

Once we pulled out onto the street, blue sky filled the moonroof. The sun burned through the windshield. My head dribbled back and forth across the headrest as we drove over the bumps. I tried to raise my seat to catch more breeze, and it slammed back down. It scared Karen. "I want to sit. Up," I explained.

"Sorry, I thought you'd be more comfortable down." She put my seat back up at the next light. Now, when I looked straight ahead, out the windshield, I felt dizzy. Karen said we should make a note of it. She pulled over and took out a pad of paper. "Dizzy?"

"I don't know." *Not dizzy, exactly.* "Not balanced." *How do you say that?* "Out of balanced."

BECKER LOG

7/5/99 3:00 p.m. "Feeling unbalanced."

It helped the dizziness if I watched the road instead of looking up. I could also scope out the bigger bumps in time to brace my head.

At last I saw the gravel of Karen's driveway.

CAREFUL WHAT YOU WISH FOR

Midafternoon on a holiday Monday. The other cars in the lot were back from Maine or the Cape. I was back from my lobotomy. I pulled my hat down and opened the car door.

"Hey, Suzy!" It was—I couldn't remember her name, a blonde, a nurse—at the door. "How're you feeling?" I waited until she advanced to the parking lot so she couldn't trap me in the walkway. She was trying to get a look under my brim.

"Hi!" My exuberance at such close range startled her.

I gripped the railing to steady myself going up the stairs. The door to Karen's place was unlocked. The air-conditioning was on. Molly trotted by me on her way to greet Karen. My ring and wallet were still on my place mat. The vial of Neurontin was where I left it. Nothing had moved.

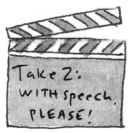

Karen stepped around me to fold down the futon-couch; the loft—no railing—was off-limits to me. "Sorry, sweetie, I didn't have time to make up the bed." She gathered all her pillows and made a big mound of them for my head.

"Thank you." It didn't matter that I didn't want to go to bed. I stepped out of my flip-flops and lay facedown. I heard Karen switch on her computer, then the "You've got mail!" and I burrowed deeper into the pillows. When I woke up, Molly was curled up on my feet.

"Catie called. She's bringing dinner."

When did the phone ring? Dinner? "What time?"

"In a few minutes, half hour tops."

No, what time is it now? *Never mind.* I remembered the VCR clock. 4:30. *Too early for dinner. Except we never had lunch. I wonder if I gained weight, lying around all day in the hospital.*

I went to the bathroom, avoiding the mirror, to weigh myself on Karen's scale.

NONTUMOR WEIGHT LOSS
(APPROXIMATE)

(PRESURGERY) 130 LBS. − (POSTSURGERY) 125 LBS. = 5 LBS.

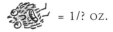 = 1/? OZ.

NONTUMOR WEIGHT LOSS = 4 LBS. 15+ OZ.

Catie was late. She had just found out that an acquaintance dropped dead onstage from a heart attack. "I'm so glad you're okay," she said.

"Mm," I agreed. *It's all relative.*

Karen and Catie talked. I nodded, drifted, interrupted once—"We forgot the pills."

Catie took advantage of the interruption to make her exit. Karen headed out to CVS. "Be back in forty-five—you'll be okay?"

I nodded and kissed her good-bye. And after she left, I found myself standing by the door again. Purposeless. Pointless. *Useless.*

PATHS FROM KAREN'S DOOR

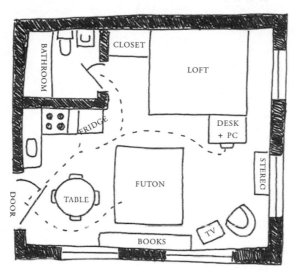

I went back to bed, rescanned the room from that angle, and decided on the bathroom. I held on to the sink for a second, afraid to see how the experience had marked my face, then pulled myself in close to the mirror and looked. My image stared back blankly. Strangely, I looked less worried. The swelling (nature's other Botox) had filled the furrow in my brow. I leaned even closer, looking for something in my eyes, some evidence of the terror, some sign *I* was inside—there was nothing.

7/5/99   7:30 p.m.   White things on face.
                     reaction to something?

The phone rang, and I let the machine pick up. I checked the VCR clock again.

How long had Karen been gone? When had she left? I couldn't remember.

I lay back down. "Brain, what do you need? . . . Brain?" No answer. Nobody home. Nothing doing. "You're scaring me."

My top lip was sticking to my teeth. I went back to the bathroom and lifted it to have a look. I had gross dentist-office-poster teeth: a plaque rim around each tooth as if I hadn't brushed in twenty years. *But I just brushed my teeth this morning.*

THE BIG H FACTOR IN PERSONAL HYGIENE

let h = hygiene *(in this case oral)* t = time
g = genetics H = health
m = labor/maintenance activities

$$h = gtmH$$

If H decreases, and g is constant,
then t and/or m must increase to maintain h.

I brushed my teeth and lifted my lip again to see what was going on now. *Lip-lifting = smiling manually. How long had it been since I smiled?* I tried. My jaw was stiff and the incision burned, but the corners of my mouth turned up. *Well, gee, there's something to smile about.*

7/5/99 8:30 p.m. Plague - right foot tingling

The doorbell buzzed. It buzzed again. I started to panic—*at the simplest thing!*—not remembering if I'd ever had to let someone in at Karen's before. I located the box by the door—it buzzed again—but I couldn't make sense of the buttons. *Just go downstairs and open the door—after you put your hat on.* The bell had rung a fourth and fifth time by the time I opened the door.

There was Karen, standing on the doormat with her arms full. "Why didn't you just buzz me in? I don't want you going up and down the stairs."

"Don't know how." She wouldn't let me help her with the groceries. I had to stop at the first landing, half a flight of stairs, to rest; she went ahead. I was barely inside when the buzzer rang again. "Like this, Suz." It was our friends Darleen and Alan.

Don't let them in! I don't want to see them! I don't want to see anybody else! I want to move to New Mexico and make all new friends. No! I want to move to New Mexico. No friends!

"You look wonderful!"

Darleen and Alan finished each other's sentences. "We were going to bring you this in the hospital, but I guess we thought you were going to be in there—I mean, it's so good that you're not—that you're okay. Anyway, this is for you. We got—Alan got a little carried away with it. . . ."

It was a box labeled "WSUZ," which held eight CDs they had made for me—recordings of my friends' get-well messages, songs, and poems.

I didn't know what to say.

After Darleen and Alan left, I took my pills, and we went to bed. Karen was holding me. "Suz, most people don't get something like that until after they're dead, for their funeral."

It wasn't just my foot; my whole right leg was tingling as we lay there. *What if I can never hike or bike or play volleyball again? What if my life is a life I don't want to live?*

I was the first one awake on Tuesday morning. I checked the VCR. Test: I tried to mouth the time. I counted up to six, three, two. *Six three two. Damn.* I waited for Karen to wake up. "What time?" I asked.

She looked at me looking at the clock. "Say it . . . please," I added.

"You try first."

 Grrr.

"Sixth—siz." Long pauses in between. "Five. Three." *Arrgh.* "Before seven."

"Six fifty-three," she says.

I repeated it, certain I'd get it once she'd said it. "Fifty-three. Sixth fifthty-three. Sixth fifty-three. Six—" *I've made her sad.* I rolled over and rubbed her forehead.

We were dozing an hour later when the phone rang. The machine picked up after the first ring; it was my dad, not sure if he had the right number. I pushed Karen out of bed, and she made a face; she was still mad at my dad.

"Alan, it's Karen, I'll get Suzy—"

My dad wanted to tell me again how relieved he was that things had gone so well.

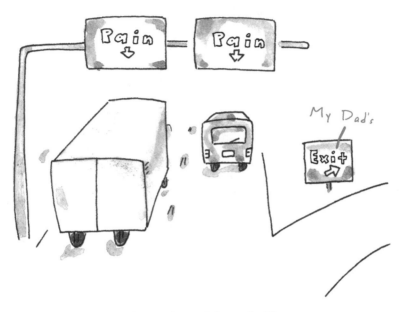

"And, what do you have planned for today?"

To Do
Poop
Take pills

To Call
Dr. Finn's office

After breakfast, Karen held out the phone. "You can call Dr. Finn any time. I don't need to be on-line or anything. . . . Why don't you call him now?"

You said ANY time.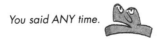

I took the phone.
"The sooner you call, the sooner we'll know what we're doing . . ."
I copied the telephone number onto a separate piece of paper, where I

could also take notes. Once again, I could not get the number to make the trip from the paper to the phone.

lousy fucking . . .

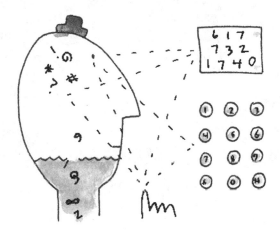

I threw the phone down on the bed. It scared Karen.

WHAT ARE YOU STARING AT?

"Want me to dial?"

I love you. "And talk."

"Sweetie, it's a brain surgery clinic; they must be used to this."

Never mind. I turned the paper sideways and wrote the number with spaces—big enough to lay a phone down in between—and dialed, moved the phone ahead, dialed . . . I got a voice-mail message, which informed me that the best way to reach the nurse was by dialing her pager, a ten-digit number followed by a five-digit ID number. I started scrawling madly, and Karen pointed to the number, already printed on the clinic card.

"Please," I was begging, "can you do it?" She took the phone, left a message, and went to work at her computer. I sat and waited by the phone.

The nurse called back within the hour. Dr. Finn wanted me to have a neuropsych evaluation—testing—to give him a clearer picture of my problems. *Does that mean he believes I have problems, or will this tell him whether I'm making them up or not?* The psychologist they had hoped would see me was on vacation, but rather than wait, they had made an appointment in two days with a colleague. She read the address slowly, waited until I was through writing it down, and then she had me read it back. "And, we have you scheduled to see Dr. Finn the next day, Friday at two-fifteen. We'll remove the stitches, and he'll have the path report."

Karen was looking at my notes. "Did you get the neuropsychologist's name?" she whispered. Too late; we had already hung up.

Nothing to do; no one to call—how many millions of times had I wished for a day like this? "Um—" I got Karen's attention without using her name— "could we go to your health club?"

She took her gym bag out of the corner. Her deodorant stick was petrified, but the guest passes in the pocket didn't have an expiration date. I borrowed a scarf—didn't want to get my good hat sweaty—put my hospital boxers back on, and waited quietly until it was time to go to the club.

Using the guest pass meant being subjected to an interview. "Suzy, right?"

I nodded.

"What's your address?"

I pointed at the address Karen had filled in at the top of the page. *Maybe I can get through the whole thing without saying anything.*

"Right, okay. So, Suzy, why are you here today?"

Because I'm not allowed to ride my bike or run: otherwise, I'd never go to a club. I'm not a sales prospect.

"Tell me a little bit about your fitness objectives."

"Recover—surgery."

"Mind my asking what kind of surgery?"

"Brain." *Ha!* I morphed before his eyes.

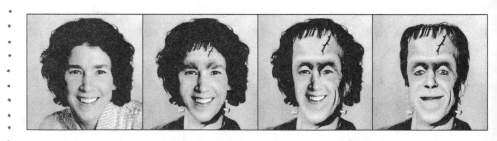

"Okay." He looked down at his clipboard, skipped to the bottom, and scribbled a signature. "Be careful out there!"

We found two incumbent bikes, side by side. I sat down, and Karen guided my feet into the stirrups. After we pedaled for twenty-five minutes, Karen helped me off the machine. My legs were no shakier than before; my head felt okay—in fact, better than okay, it was worth noting.

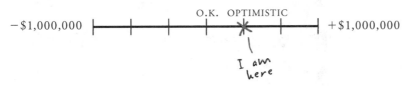

HOW ARE YOU FEELING?

$-\$1,000,000$ ——————— O.K. OPTIMISTIC ——————— $+\$1,000,000$

I am here

I can train for Ride FAR on a machine until I can get back on my—

7/6/99 4:30 p.m. Right index finger trembling

More accurately, waving uncontrollably. I held it up to show Karen and then dropped it back down to my side. It kept waving and then stopped, just as suddenly, when we were changing into our bathing suits.

I was still wearing the scarf and now Karen's suit, the straps cinched with my sneaker shoelace. I didn't mind being seen in it, I just wouldn't want to be recognized. . . .

"You never come here!" It was one of Karen's friends; she laughed at Karen. "And you, how are *you* doing?" She sat down on the edge of the whirlpool.

My shoulders were up around my ears, in part to keep my body from drifting away from the wall of the pool. "Okay."

Karen explained about my speech, and her friend smiled knowingly. "It's one of those life-changing experiences." Her scars flashed into focus. She had been flung through a windshield in high school. She knew how badly I wanted to rewind, do over. I felt lucky. Not luckier than her, just lucky to have run into her my first full day out of the hospital.

I took another nap when we got back to Karen's, and then I tried writing again. "Spell *forgiving* for me?"

Karen handed me the dictionary. I used to love looking things up: not just new words, but the exact definition of an old word, or finding words I never knew existed, odd pairings of guide words, or studying the pictures—why *beret*, not *bergamot?* The dictionary sat flattening my thighs. *You can't look something up if you can't spell it.* I moved the dictionary on to the bed and repeated the question. She started to spell it. "Write it?"

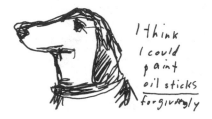

I think
I could
paint
oil sticks
forgivingly

All th words I used to find in the dictionary.

Karen was through working. I closed my notebook. "What do you want to have for dinner?" she asked. Cooking wasn't an option. She uses her enamel stove top as a display for little things she's collected, some that I've given her.

"Popcorn," I answered, as in "movies and." The thought of reading a menu and ordering out loud made me queasy. We agreed on something summery, *Notting Hill,* with Julia Roberts and Hugh Grant.

There were long stretches, watching that movie, where I felt okay—sitting in the dark, holding Karen's hand, following the plot—where for the first time I actually felt normal. It had been only a few days, but they were long days. *How many does it take before you forget what normal feels like?*

That night, we switched sides of the bed so I could hold Karen without lying on my incision. I lay awake, staring at the back of her head. Someone once introduced us as "two independent, artistic, funny women." My dad described it as my first truly democratic relationship. Now that I had less of a voice, I wondered if democracy was the best form of relationship for me. Maybe I'd be better off where words weren't so important, where I was accepted, not challenged all the time.

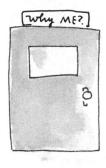

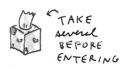

The next morning Karen announced, "Suz, I have stuff I need to do today, a bunch of errands...."

"Mm."

Can't be sitting around taking care of me all day.

I'd hoped we could go to the health club.

"Do you want to go to the health club when I get back?"

"That's okay."

"That's okay?"

That's okay as in NO! I don't want to go to the health club. I don't want anything zero zip zilch nada from you!

"Let—see," I stuttered.

She shook her head, exasperated. I lay back down. The phone rang. This morning it was my mother on the machine. "I know Karen's taking good care of you, but I *am* your mother. If there's anything I can do, let me know. I love you. Bye-bye." Click.

"Can you call?" I asked Karen.

"Your mother?"

I nodded.

"You'll talk?"

I nodded again. She handed me the phone.

"Mommy, Suzy." She asked how I was. "Good—Can I go to your club?—We went yesterday—I'm fine."

She'd offered me her guest pass a hundred times before, and I'd never gone. "I promised that guest pass to your father." *My father?!*

Is he planning a visit?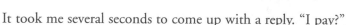

It took me several seconds to come up with a reply. "I pay?"

"Oh, that's all right. I should be able to get another pass out of them." My mother would come get me, and Karen would pick me up later.

Karen was on her way out. "Don't forget your pills with lunch."

"Not today."

She checked. "Two milligrams every six hours: breakfast, lunch, dinner, and bedtime."

"Less today."

"It *is* less." She brought the paper over. "Yesterday you were taking three milligrams, *three* pills four times a day."

No, yesterday, as a matter of fact, I was taking one *pill to reduce the swelling—the probable cause of my speech impediment—four times a day.* I had never checked the milligrams.

I am not fit to take care of myself.

Karen called Dr. Finn's office: three pills the remaining three times today, two beginning tomorrow. She redrew the chart.

Pill Taking for DUMMIES

	WED	THUR	FRI	SAT
Decadron (TAPER)	● ● ● ⊠ ☐ ☐ ☐	● ● ☐ ☐ ☐ ☐	● ☐ ☐ ☐ ☐	● ☐ ☐ ☐ ☐

That night after we got back from my mother's, the photographs Karen had taken at the hospital were sitting on my place mat. I flipped through them once. Karen said I could keep the doubles. I didn't want them. Photographs can be so inaccurate. Everyone, including me, looked like they were having a good time.

IT was
BRAIN SURGERY

I was looking forward to the testing. I dressed in my last clean shirt, blue chambray with buttons, my black shorts, and my hat, which could have passed for a fashion statement since the temperature had dropped.

The neuropsychologist's outfit made me feel like I was still wearing a hospital johnny.

POWER DRESSING 101
WITH DEBORAH KNIGHT

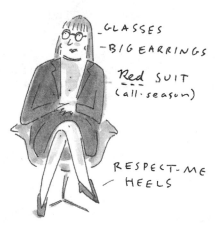

- GLASSES
- BIG EARRINGS

Red SUIT
(all·season)

RESPECT-ME
HEELS

Her office was dark. The blinds were drawn, and her desk lamp stuck to its job description.

"When did you start having seizures?" she asked.

> Behavioral observation: Ms. Becker presented as a somewhat anxious woman who was noticeably concerned about the difficulties she was experiencing.

"Nineteen nineteen." *1995.* "Nine. Five. No. Four years ago."

After a pathetic rendition of my medical history, I handed her copies of my cat book and fellowship application, some evidence of my former self. Before Dr. Knight had had a chance to look at the work, Karen volunteered that I was a very bright and talented woman. It sounded better coming from her, but she wasn't exactly an unbiased source.

Dr. Knight asked Karen about my difficulties. "She stutters, although"—Karen adjusted her right sleeve, her deadpan giveaway—"she's always had a tendency to mumble."

> Her partner also noted that she stutters occasionally, though she noted that she always had a tendency to mumble.

Dr. Knight handed the cat book back without saying a word.

"How many copies has that book sold, Suz?" Karen asked. She didn't wait for me to answer. "It was a *New York Times* bestseller. . . . Number one. Million—"

"That book?" Dr. Knight turned to me. "I'd like to keep your application folder."

I nodded. "Um—I'm afraid I can't do it."

"Have a baby?" She had leafed through the book project proposal. "I don't think you should rule it out yet."

WHAT'S ON THE TABLE

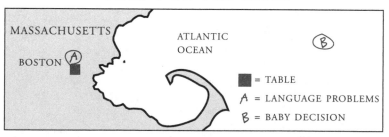

Yet. Yet? *Yetyetyetyetyetyetyetyetyetyetyetyet—are you suggesting I might not be mentally capable of having children?!*

I couldn't stop crying. Karen rubbed the back of my neck. Deborah Knight waited for me to pull myself together.

"Can we get started?" she asked. "I think she'll be better off alone for the testing." She opened the door for Karen. Then she pulled a large binder off her bookshelf and wheeled a chair over to another table. I wheeled my chair over beside her.

She was motivated to perform well and cooperated with the evaluation.

"Each of these pages has a picture," she explained once she was seated. "I'm going to ask you to identify the picture. For example"—she turned the notebook inside out and stood it on the table—"if I showed you this picture . . .

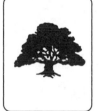

I'd feel like I was in first grade.

. . . you'd say *tree.*"

I blanked on *yoke,* third to last, and there were a few others I got in a roundabout way:

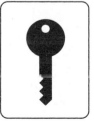

"Thing for a lock, to unlock." But I finished within the allotted time, and I was feeling encouraged. Night Nurse would have been impressed.

Dr. Knight wheeled her chair away from the table; we were going off-binder. "Can you recite the alphabet?"

At this point, I knew better than to say yes without thinking. Nothing came to mind. I invoked my visual memory: I could see pairs of letters—capital and lowercase—lined up above a blackboard, but I couldn't zoom in to read them. *Maybe if I stop thinking altogether: A-B-C—maybe if I sing it: A-B-C-D-E-F-G;* I couldn't untangle *L-M-N-O-P.*

"Time." She made a notation. "Now I'd like you to recite it backwards," as if I'd had no problem reciting it forwards. As if the slightest hint of empathy would have invalidated my results.

I closed my eyes; the room, the blackboard, and the letters above it were spinning. I closed my eyes tighter—"Z-L-X, no—" *Wait, I can see.* "Z, Wha." *What a joke.*

> She was teary at times, especially when she perceived she was having difficulties.

I shook my head.

"Now I'd like you to name the months of the year, beginning with January."

"January . . . January . . ." I could have been repeating the end of the question instead of beginning the answer.

> She tended to want to respond to questions quickly.

I named all twelve months in seven seconds on the eighth try. Then she wanted me to say them backwards. The word *backwards* had the same dizzying effect. Twelve months, backwards, twenty-two seconds. I lost count of the number of tries.

"Can you name the days of the week?"

Can. Could. Did, only *Thursday* came out instead of *Tuesday* at first. She gave me a "very good" on that one.

Word generation: "When I tell you to begin, I want you to name as many *A* words, words that start with the letter *A,* as you can. You may begin now."

"Apple." *Ass. Asshole. Ass ass ass ass ass.*

Working memory: "I am going to read you a series of numbers. When I am through, I'd like you to repeat them back to me. The sequences will increase in length and difficulty; listen carefully, and try to remember as many numbers as you can. . . ."

Simple word problems: "Do two pounds of flour weigh more than one pound?"

Deborah Knight went to pick up her daughter and left me alone to self-administer the reading, writing, and grammar tests (under the surveillance of her assistant). I was unable to finish the reading test in the time allowed. New personal worst. The writing test was fill in the blank. If I had to pick a test, this one most closely approximated what I used to do. You were supposed to write the middle sentence in the style of the other two. I stared and stared at the blank until it reversed out when I looked up at the wall. *Forget about the right answer, then—put something funny.* That's how I'd always gotten myself out of these situations in the past.

"Time." It was the assistant. "Last one." She placed the grammar test in front of me.

There was no sign of her when I finished. I was free to leave, I supposed, but maybe not—maybe there was a one-way mirror somewhere. I sat there with my hands on my hat and studied the picture of Deborah Knight with her daughter on the desk. *Have you ever tried to imagine what it feels like not to ace these tests?*

Like crying. Let me make that into a complete sentence: It makes me feel like crying. Like breaking something, like breaking everything in your office, like whipping that fat notebook against the wall until all the fucking pages fall out all over the floor.

Karen was waiting in the lobby. She stood up. There were papers from her book-in-progress fanned out on the floor around her feet. She held out her arms to gather me in. "Hurry," I said. "Please. I want to go."

We were in the car before we spoke again. Karen said, "It was awful. I'm so sorry, sweetie."

I couldn't answer. I just cried. A couple of blocks from the hospital, the color red caught my eye. Dr. Knight was hurrying, in her sneakers, to pick up her daughter.

"Isn't that—?" I pointed and Karen spotted her.

"You should go," I said after I stopped crying. "And I will call when I know how I am."

"I'll be home Saturday, Suz. I'll only be gone thirty-six hours—I can stay if you want, and go to Dr. Finn's—"

"No. I mean leave me. You should leave. I cannot be a partner. It's not—I'm not who you loved. You should be with someone—"

"I am *not* leaving. What kind of person would leave? You wouldn't leave me—I love you, Suz. We're going to get through this."

"I don't know—I don't know how I will be. We haven't even been one whole year." *Listen to me, the way I sound.* "I will call, and if you're not with anyone—"

"Stop. Stop saying that."

I couldn't watch her cry. I leaned the seat back, and we didn't talk again for thirty miles.

"Are you looking forward to being home?" Karen asked at the exit.

I was. I was looking forward to seeing my animals and my garden. To being alone. I didn't say that; she must have been thinking the same thing.

We rounded the last curve before my driveway, and for a second, it was so vivid—I could see myself driving in the opposite direction, one week ago. I was *so* fine. Naïve.

It seemed as if I'd been gone much longer, the way everything needed attention. The lawn needed mowing. The house needed painting. All of a sudden, it seemed so big. *Will I be able to take care of this place? Will I be able to take care of myself?*

Someone had planted the window boxes. Portulaca—about all there was left this late in the season—a scraggly substitute for my geraniums, cascading lobelia, and sweet alyssum. *You are so ungrateful.*

Mister greeted me inside the door.

"Careful of your head, Suz," Karen cautioned.

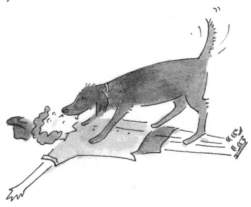

Robin emerged from the other room as if it were her home. I walked into the kitchen and was distracted by the things that were askew, *almost in their right places.* Robin saw me surveying the room. "Everybody's shedding," she apologized. "I swear, I swept this morning."

She shouldn't be apologizing. I rearranged the bowls on the shelves. *I am ungrateful* and *unappreciative.* I put the glasses back in their rows. *I will go to Hell.* I opened the refrigerator; there was oven-fried chicken, potato salad, and deviled eggs. Our favorite summer picnic as kids.

"And she made brownies," Robin said. My mother had brought dinner, but she wouldn't stay. She was afraid she'd say the wrong thing.

After dinner, I was transferred to Robin's custody. Karen went over the discharge instructions with my pill chart, and she showed Robin how to put on a bandage when I went out. (I'd started going bandageless in private.) She asked one last time if I wanted her to go to Dr. Finn's. "Promise to call as soon as you know anything?"

What about our 11 p.m. call?

Or am I just your patient now? Forget it.

"Call when you get there?" I wouldn't have made myself ask if it weren't for the night driving. She promised, and gave her customary *beep-beep* as she drove down the driveway.

Robin had finished the dishes and was watching TV in the living room. I wandered from room to room, hoping to feel at home again, hoping the rooms' memories would take over, bring me back.

An hour and a half later, Karen called; she'd made it. I took Mister out and said good night to Robin. "Thank you, Rob."

"I'm glad I can do this for you, Suz."

Mister followed me up the stairs and staked out his side of the bed, a generous half when Karen and Molly were gone. The room was cool; night air moved through the window. I put away a pile of clothes that Robin had washed and folded, and got into bed.

SLEEPING in my OWN BED

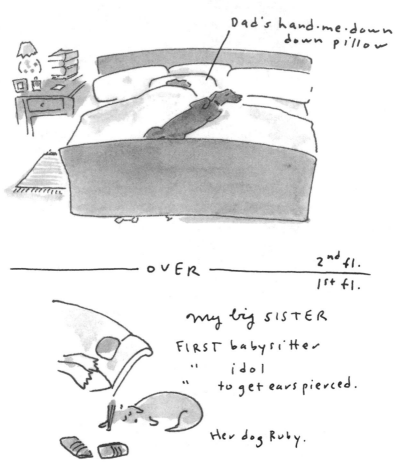

Dad's hand·me·down
down pillow

———— OVER ———— 2nd fl.
1st fl.

my big SISTER

FIRST babysitter
"   idol
"   to get ears pierced.

Her dog Ruby.

Friday morning I woke up before Mister and checked the clock—I still couldn't say the time. *Please, give me a break.* . . . Temporary amnesia, a few minutes of waking forgetfulness—a reprieve. I shuffled Mister by the guest room so as not to wake Robin or her dog on the way down. He stood in the kitchen, looking up at me, wagging his tail expectantly: Walk me, feed me, talk to me, c'mon, what're you waiting for?

"You want dinner—breakfast?" I watched him while he ate. He *was* the perfect practice audience.

"Wanna go out, bady? . . . Bay-bee?" *All the things I used to say without thinking. . . .*

Mister went to his morning spot, the mudroom trough, in the old attached barn off the kitchen. I gardened right outside his window. After five years, it was still a beginner's garden—gaudy and overcrowded, the result of my impatience and distrust during the weeks before the first show of color.

I turned the soil with my scuffle hoe. The dark brown overtook the sun-dried light brown. The new earth smelled damp. When I finished hoeing, I pulled the suckers off the tomato plants, checked the snap peas, which were almost ready for picking, and deadheaded my flowers. I saved cutting a bouquet for last.

I held the scissors in my hand and awaited some sort of command: *How long? How many?* I tried visual recall, an old bouquet—something for the jelly jar or the small white pitcher. . . . *Nothing.* I set the scissors down on the blue table by the kitchen door.

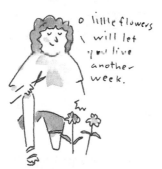

ACT of
SELF-
RESTRAINT

O little flowers
will let
you live
another
week.

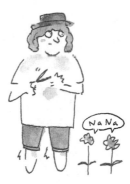

ACT of
SELF
RESTRAINED

NaNa

I swept the paths, watered the annuals, and went back inside to make coffee. None of my movements felt fluid, but some, I noted, after repetition, back in my own place, were beginning to feel familiar. Others— cutting flowers, making coffee—things you need a "feel" for, were not.

I blamed my brain. Not the motor controls— the connection to the requisite knowledge or memory was down.

I carried a weak cup of coffee up to my office. The place was eerily neat. My chair was rolled in; the desks were cleared. The answering machine was blinking silently on top of the filing cabinet. Deborah Knight's evaluation was on top of a pile of faxes. I picked it up, left everything else exactly as it was, and went back downstairs.

Robin and I read the evaluation at the kitchen table. I fixated on the mistakes *Ha!* she made in my medical history. *Ha! Ha! Ha!*

Robin read ahead: "Suz, do two pounds of flour weigh more than one pound?"

I recognized the question. "Say it again."

"She said you had mild difficulties with the complex comprehension of ideational material, such as 'Do two pounds . . .'"

The evaluation listed my raw test scores, but there were no means, charts, or normal curves for comparison. Overall, Dr. Knight summarized, my scores were in the high average to superior range—*Is that on a scale where "Is two more than one?" equals complex ideational material?*—with a few notable exceptions.

> ### Things You Need a Feel For
>
> Handwriting
> Drawing
> Making wire animals
> Phone-dialing
> Typing
> Shooting a basketball
> Setting a volleyball
> Playing the flute
> Massage
> Sex
> Giving a cat
> subcutaneous fluids
> Sewing
> Adjusting an antenna

She had relative difficulties on the writing subtests though I wonder if these were relative weaknesses in the past as I have reviewed her previous writing.

Where were you at career counseling time?

The relatively strong scores—a 97 in spelling, 81 in reading comprehension—actually made me feel worse.

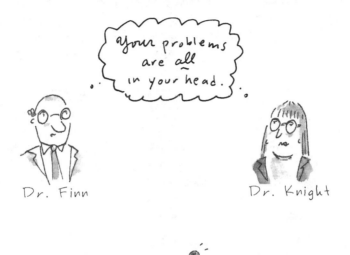

Dr. Finn   Dr. Knight

TERRY GROSS: You *really* didn't like this woman.

ME: Deborah Knight? She's probably better than I remember. It's convenient to be able to focus all your anger on one person.

TG: It made me curious—do you have to worry about a lawsuit when you write a book like this?

ME: I changed her name. Her real name is Sheila Day. I worry more about the people who wouldn't sue me, like my family—it was hard to leave their imperfections in.

Meredith drove me to my appointment with Dr. Finn the next day. There were refreshments out, a festive touch—the difference between the regular office hours and the Friday "Brain Tumor Clinic." Katondra bellowed a big, "Suzy Becker, Suzy Becker! Look at you—I knew you'd do great!" I forgot to object and smiled up at her from under my hat.

One of Dr. Finn's nurses greeted Meredith and me, and she pointed me out to another woman behind the reception desk as she took us back.

"Everyone loves your book, Suzy. So, how're you doing?"

"Okay."

"You still—listen to me, *still*—it's been what, a week, right?—having trouble with your speech? He didn't touch your sense of humor, did he? I'll kill him!"

I didn't answer; I couldn't bring myself to smile even though she'd earned one. *Yes, he did. My sense of humor—my career, my personality, my coping mechanism—*

Donna sat us down in a couple of chairs. "Listen, I have husbands who—hey, where's your partner—Karen, isn't it?" She looked at Meredith. "Are you a sister?" Meredith nodded. "Older or younger?"

"Younger," Meredith answered. "Karen went to Maine."

"Anyway," Donna went on, "I have husbands who come in and sit across from me, here, with their wives who just had surgery, and they ask me, 'When am I going to get my wife back?' and I look at them and say, 'Your wife's right there. You better take good care of her.' But, I know what they mean." She paused. "You had brain surgery. If you had knee surgery, you wouldn't expect to be feeling so hunky-dory, right? Give it four weeks. I'm talking a month of R and R, rest and relaxation— let other people, Karen, your sister here, take care of you. Pamper yourself. See what I'm saying?" She looked at Meredith. "Right?"

Recovery Clock

4 weeks

She inspected my incision. The stitches were ready to come out. "You all set with your medications now, no more problems?"

I showed her the chart Karen set up according to the discharge instructions and pointed to 7/10, the next day. "Last day," I said.

"Let me see that—no, no, you keep tapering these off: four milligrams tomorrow, three for a couple of days, two." She revised the chart as she talked. "You don't want to stop taking those little pills. Places where they don't have them, they don't put the skull back together. Can't. They leave the hole, and the brain kind of bulges out there until the swelling goes down." She looked to make sure the story had sunk in. "Let me see if I can't find Dr. Finn."

"She's nice," Meredith said after she left. "Everybody is. Must be kind of depressing to work here. . . ."

The nurse came back without Dr. Finn. "He's going to be a while. You want to talk to someone. Psychologist? Psychiatrist? We have 'em all here, and we like to keep 'em busy. Seriously, they know what you're going through; it could help. Should I?"

I nodded.

She sent the psychiatrist in. Meredith started to stand, but I pressed her forearm back down toward the arm of her chair. Dr. Saxon pulled up a third chair. He leaned back with his hands in the opened-prayer position.

The Opened-Prayer Position

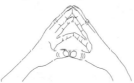

(a.k.a. Spider Doing
Push-ups on Mirror)

"How are you feeling, Suzy?"
    "Scared—about my speech."
    "You sound pretty good to me."

If I hear that one more time...

"Can I say something, Suz?" Meredith looked Dr. Saxon in the eye and said, "She does *not* sound pretty good. She is having trouble putting two sentences together. She has a hard time explaining what she does. She's speaking very slowly, for her. . . . She does not sound like herself."

"She's had brain surgery," Dr. Saxon counseled; neither of us responded. He opened my folder. "Why don't you tell me what you do?"

"I write books—I do art. The art—"

"You illustrate your own books."

"Yes." He was waiting for more. "I do Ride FAR."

"Uh-huh. Let me ask you something else. Have you ever had to deal with disappointment before?"

Is there a thirty-six-year-old alive who hasn't?

DISAPPOINTMENT TIMELINE (*PARTIAL*)

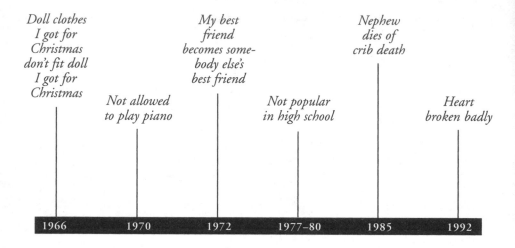

Doll clothes I got for Christmas don't fit doll I got for Christmas

My best friend becomes somebody else's best friend

Nephew dies of crib death

Not allowed to play piano

Not popular in high school

Heart broken badly

| 1966 | 1970 | 1972 | 1977–80 | 1985 | 1992 |

He was still looking at me, his eyebrows still raised.

"Yes," I answered.

He offered to write me a prescription for anti-depressants. *Is that your diagnosis? I don't want some pills to make me happy like this; I want someone to help me get my self back.*

After several excruciating minutes of silence, Dr. Saxon concluded I was through talking and handed me his card in case I wanted to see him again.

It wasn't long before Dr. Finn came in to see us. He wanted to know how the speech was coming. "You're telling me you used to be a real motormouth, huh?"

It wasn't that I used to be a motormouth, it's just—at least I used to have a choice. I could talk if I felt like it.

"How's the artwork?"

I showed him the sketches I'd done in the hospital. "I have no ideas," I said, before he could say anything.

"Tell me more about that."

> Effects on brain function are often subtle but nonetheless potentially devastating.
>
> —JOHN SAXON,
> *BRAIN CANCERS*

July 5, 1999

I could see he was concerned: I wanted to be able to explain it—the only words I could come up with were, "I lost my impulse."

"You think I took that away?"

"I'm not myself." That was my fallback.

"Well"—he was leaning forward, looking up at me over his glasses, under my brim—"I'm talking to *somebody*." He said it so lightly. "Some part of you is still here. . . ."

"Fith. Hath. Half."

He leaned back. "Dr. Knight's preliminary assessment *did* show some impairment—you need to give it some time. Everybody's brain is organized a little differently—some of the pathways have been disrupted, but they will repair themselves or the neurons will find new pathways. I have complete confidence your brain will heal itself. Give it a month. Why not take a vacation for a few weeks?"

"Ride FAR," I answered.

"Can't you get somebody else to take care of the bike ride? And listen, if you decide to do speech therapy," he cautioned, "don't get frustrated by it—that won't do you any good. Get up and walk out if you want."

He took out the pathology report. I got my pencil ready.

"The tissue was fine."

"Benign?" Meredith asked.

"It was a gliosis, a sort of scar tissue we don't see much of, not actually a tumor at all."

Luck

"A scar from what?" Meredith asked.

"We don't know, but it's not the kind of thing, once we remove it, that grows back." He turned to me. "I want to see you in three weeks. We'll have another look at an MRI—things should be pretty well cleared up by then. Meantime"—he was trying to catch my eye again—"let people help you. It can be a valuable experience. . . . Is there anything else?"

I didn't want to keep a roomful of people with *real* tumors waiting. "Can I bike?"

"I think you should do whatever you feel like doing. Within reason. If you feel like you can ride a bike—I'm sure I don't have to tell you to wear a helmet—and that's going to make you feel good"—he shrugged—"then I think you should do it."

"Thank—you."

The nurse stayed to take the stitches out. She handed me my hat. "I know he told you to do whatever you want. I'm going to tell you to be real careful. You don't want to fall on your head before it's all back together again. And between now and"—she'd lost track of the month—"and September, you're at increased risk for a seizure. You rest, Suzy; let people take care of you. Treat you like a princess. You get to be princess for a month, tell Karen I said so, hm? Okay, you can put your hat back on." I hadn't felt a thing. "I'm going to say it one more time: Give it a month."

I would give it a month. Something in me uncoiled.

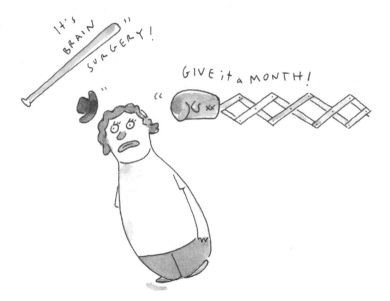

Meredith and I stopped at the supermarket on the way home. I had a list of ingredients I needed to buy for bran muffins and dinner for Karen on Saturday. I like to go shopping, the way some people like to vacuum. My shopping list is organized to help me navigate the aisles; then I usually use a kind of comparison shopping—buy the cheapest kind that meets the quality standard—to navigate the brands. But I couldn't do the math, and I was too embarrassed (by my frugality, not my deficit) to ask Meredith to do the math for me. *What's a few more dollars, princess?*

I spotted a neighbor rounding the aisle, rolling her cart toward us. Margaret and her daughter—her daughter_____. She was working the opposite side of the aisle; we had a chance to slip by, but I needed Meredith's cooperation. "Mer." I wasn't loud, just panicky. She whipped around as if maybe I'd fallen down or was having a seizure. "Neighbor!"

The neighbor had seen us. Now I'd lost her name, too. "Hi! Hi!" The second "hi" was in place of her name, although it could've been for the daughter. Meredith had her back to us, studying the shelves.

"Suzy, how are you? Are you ever around? Stan and I keep wanting to have you over, but I never see your car. We're home this weekend. Maybe Sunday? I'll call you, listen—I like that hat!" She rolled by. I was all jittery, as if I'd almost been in a car accident.

At the register, I had already run my ATM card through more times than there were possible stripe-orientations. The cashier took the card. "Credit or debit?"

I don't know. Neither? The hat trapped the heat from my head. "ATM."

She hit a button and slid the card and looked off toward the produce section. "Punch in your code."

I pointed my finger. . . . The memory was gone. *I wish big bolts would pop out of my neck. I need some kind of a sign or a button.* Meredith was shielding me from all the stares. She paid and we left.

I hadn't gotten over the transaction by the time we got to the house. I walked right by Robin and set the bags down. "Is she okay?" I heard Robin ask Meredith as she walked through the door. *No, she can't use a bank card.*

"It's benign!" Meredith answered, and they hugged each other. I put the groceries away while they called my parents. Meredith dialed the phone, and I left a message for Karen.

Robin had started to set the table. I moved a new bouquet of get-well

flowers over to the counter; the smell of lilies, magnified by my medications, made me feel sick. I looked back at the table and counted three
places. "Meredith staying?"

"No." She paused, hoping I'd remember. "Laura's coming."

That's right. I hadn't been able to put off her visit any longer.

After dinner, Robin insisted on doing the dishes so Laura and I could
have time alone. I didn't want time alone. I didn't want Laura to see me
without my speech in the first place. I stood by the sink. "Why don't you
make your muffins?" Robin suggested.

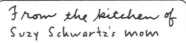

From the kitchen of
Suzy Schwartz's mom

Tried 'n' True Poo-poo Muffins
Makes 24 muffins

They're #1
for #2!

3 cups 100% All Bran
2 cups bran flakes
5 ½ cups whole wheat flour
2 ½ cups sugar
4 teaspoons cinnamon
Raisins, craisins, blueberries, bananas (optional)

3 teaspoons baking soda
1 quart buttermilk
4 eggs
1 cup safflower oil
½ cup molasses

Mix all the ingredients in a large bowl. Refrigerate the batter
for 6 to 8 hours before baking at 350° F in greased tins.

I took out my Texas muffin tin and gave Laura the job of greasing it. I
set the oven and opened the bran. *One quarter of three?* I asked my brain.
"Fractions? HA! No way!"

I asked the question out loud. Robin repeated the question, spelling-
bee style, preparing to answer it. "One is one quarter of four." She was
showing her work. "Three quarters is one quarter of three." Laura agreed.
The same math worked for two cups of bran flakes. When I got to the
whole wheat flour, she slowed down.

Laura, who can be quiet, especially when one of my sisters is around, piped up, "First you have to make an improper fraction." That sounded familiar. "Eleven halves times one quarter. Eleven eighths. One and three eighths." I poured the flour in the measuring cup: *Is 1⅜ cups of flour more than 1½ cups of flour?*

Laura painted my toenails while the muffins baked.* Red, green, blue, and silver. We were silent while we both concentrated on my toes. I used to love to watch my mother polish her nails on Saturday nights, hypnotized by the brush fanning the enamel across the nail, and the smell. I still like the smell.

Laura left me with my feet propped up. "My dad," she said, "would be happy to answer any questions or talk to you about any of this. . . .

Isn't your dad the one that got me into all this?

And I'd be happy to help, y'know, with Ride FAR or whatever. . . ." She let herself out.

Robin had gone upstairs. Mister took Laura's place on the couch. We dozed while my toes dried, waiting for the oven timer to ring. I left the muffins cooling and put the rest of the house to bed.

I lay on my back on top of the covers. Mister's back and tail ran the length of me. *I'll give it a month. I will. Even if a thousand neurosurgeons couldn't have predicted . . . what are my choices?*

---

* Recipe Police: I know the directions say to refrigerate the batter, but I had brain surgery . . . and they turned out fine.

CRÈME BRÛLÉE

I spent most of Saturday making dinner for Karen, her summer favorite: hamburgers, sliced tomatoes, homemade coleslaw, lemonade, fresh corn, and key lime pie. I turned the radio on, then turned it right back off. Cooking, I'd forgotten, now required my undivided attention.

Karen was thrilled with the meal. And aside from my new clumsiness (I had a small tantrum when the ejected beaters plummeted to the bottom of the key lime custard) or the fact that it took all afternoon and part of an evening to make a hamburger dinner, I was satisfied with the results. The time apart had done us good.

The next morning, Robin packed up to leave. She wouldn't let me help her with her bags. When I followed her outside to say good-bye, she stopped at my car. "Suz, I replaced that brake light and had your oil changed."

I hugged her, watched her pull down the drive, then went back to bed. Karen and I made love. It meant more to her than dinner. Months later, a couples therapist would tell us how people who have had heart attacks, life-threatening illness, or accidents often don't want to make love for some period of time. They have the feeling (it's normal, although in most cases inaccurate) that it will kill them. I didn't think it was going to kill me, but a series of small explosions along the pathways couldn't be good for the rebuilding project. And it made me acutely aware of all of my shortcomings. So began the Lovers' Catch-22: Karen needed to make love to feel loved. I needed to feel loved to make love . . .

Karen bought the Sunday paper, and we spent the rest of the afternoon in the backyard. She read, and I alternated resting on the lawn furniture and resting on the blanket in the grass with trips inside for lemonade or more pillows.

Monday, July 12: I'd been out of the hospital for one week. Karen left for work by 8:30, a fresh start after two months of neglect. Two months and ten days (to be exact) since I'd had the telltale seizure. I went up to my office—not "back to work"—to see if there was anything that required my immediate attention.

To Do	To Call
Fellowship registration	Pelvic ultrasound
Check e-mail	Therapist
Send training ride info	Vet
	Cancel TV appearance:
	Creatively Speaking

The therapist was relieved to hear from me. She made time to see me the next day. "Are you okay to drive?" (She wasn't asking if it was legal.) The question hadn't occurred to me, or anybody else—I *had* to be.

"Mister!" I went to whistle. Some puckery air came out—it was either the swelling or my mouth—*oh, never mind.* "Let's go!" *Let's find out if I can drive.*

My car sits low, and I was sitting low in my car, slumped. My head was too heavy to hold up straight. I drove a mile on the back road to the highway; then I tried a few miles of four-lane. My left hand in the ten o'clock position, an anti-rightward-listing stabilizer; my right hand at twelve I used as a fulcrum when I raised myself to check the rearview mirror. I turned around at the first exit; I was fine—not up to city driving or parallel parking, but good enough for a trip to the therapist's before Karen came back to get me.

Mister and I walked around the reservoir on the way home. Bright
blue sky. Myriad shades of green leaves. The brown-green water flecked
with spots of pure white light. Everything looked more brilliant. Imbued
with independence. Or convalescence. Or medication . . . *Who cares?! Give
me a million days of gray!* My old self never would've said "who cares" to
the sun—*AND my speech back!*

How Many Dog Miles in One Human Mile?

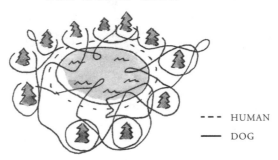

- - - HUMAN

—— DOG

I wandered up to my office again and turned on my computer to re-
trieve my e-mail. I deleted a third of the messages without even opening them. If I read ten each day for the next six days (forgetting to take new
mail into account), I'd be caught up by the weekend. I opened the first one
from someone who had cc'ed me on a message she had sent her first-year
business school students; she thought my surgery made an inspiring post-
script to the guest lecture on entrepreneurship I'd given back in March. It
made me feel slightly sick. Seeing my address, which she had included in
the e-mail, also reminded me I had a post office box I needed to check.
How much of the rest of my life am I forgetting?

I hit REPLY and stared at the monitor, waiting for my thoughts to
liquid-crystallize on the screen. CANCEL. *Make that five e-mails a day.*

I started a list for Karen.

Just then the mail truck came barreling up the driveway, honking.
Special delivery. I hurried downstairs and out through the garden. "How
are ya?" The woman's voice had the same timbre as her honk.

"Okay," I said, signing for the package.

"Just okay? What's wrong?"

I pointed. "My lawn?" She'd pulled up to the garden fence over two truck-lengths of grass. *Lawn* was a stretch, considering the weedy state it was in.

"Oh well, *excuse me!*" She barreled off.

My agent had sent me crème brûlée on dry ice. It was a healing omen.

Healing Statements for Surgery

Patient's Name Suzy Becker

(Give this page to your surgeon and another to your anesthesiologist. Tape a third page to your hospital gown so it is visible as you go into surgery.)

As I am going under the anesthesia, please say:

#1 "Following the operation, you will feel comfortable and you will heal very well." (Repeat 5 times.)

After saying the statements, please put on my earphones and start my tape player.

Toward the end of surgery, remove my earphones. Say:

#2 "Your operation has gone very well." (Repeat 5 times.)

#3 "Following this operation, you will be hungry for crème brûlée."

"You will be thirsty and you will urinate easily." (Repeat 5 times.)

There were still hours until dinner. Hours after that until bed. I wandered around like a ghost in my house: *what to do, what to do . . .*

I remembered the TV, which lives in the living room closet. I opened the door, sat down, and watched my very first *Oprah!*

Her guest was talking and talking—I was riveted by his mouth. *I want his mouth. I want all of the words coming out of his mouth.*

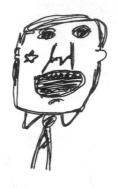

Remember:
#1. It is a
Compassionate
universe.

Compassionate universe. Ha! I shut him off and walked out to the barn. Maybe I'd mow the lawn. I rolled the mower out onto the driveway. Just looking at the starter was enough to set off the intracranial pressure alarm. I rolled it back in.

Ask for HELP.

Who am I supposed to ask? Karen can't start a lawn mower. I can't ask someone to drive out to Bolton just to start a mower. I suppose I *could* ask my neighbor, the one I saw at the grocery store. The word was going to get out anyway. *Who cares—publish it in the paper! At least that way I won't have to go around explaining myself.*

I rehearsed the question on my way over. The husband opened the door. "Hey, Stan!" Stan's the president (and the youngest member) of Bolton's Lions Club.

"Suzy! Margaret said she just bumped into you!"

"Mm." *So what if this is a non sequitur.* "Can you starp"—*Start start, I mean start*—"my mower?"

"Of course," he said without a second's hesitation.

"Nn I had brain surgery," I announced once we had the mower back out, and pointed to my hat. I couldn't help being blunt.

"Gosh." It took him a few seconds. "You okay?"

"Going to be."

He yanked the starter, and the engine drowned out the possibility of any further conversation. I gave him a thumbs-up and a wave, and he headed back down the driveway.

Halfway through the front yard, I walked into my second tree. It was the brim-obstructed view. A twig impaled my hat, not far from the incision, and I let go of the mower, which promptly stalled. *Enough.* I rolled the mower back into the barn.

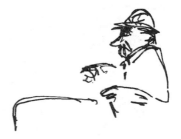

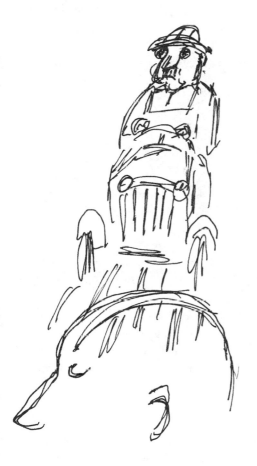

If I feel physically as if the top of my head were taken off, I know that is poetry.

Emily Dickinson

The next morning, I went back to my computer and drafted a reminder about the fifty-mile training ride coming up on Saturday. My fingers had forgotten the keyboard. *One more thing.* By the time I had hunted-and-pecked out a word, I'd lost the sentence. After two hours, I resorted to cutting and pasting from an old reminder. I forwarded the message to Meredith for one last look before sending it out, and she went over it with me, line by line. There were transposed letters, extra spaces, and a misspelling—big blind spots in my proofreading vision. More holes shot in my confidence.

She stayed on the phone until I'd made the last change. I looked at my watch: two and a half hours with corrections. *Give yourself credit for sticking with it* . . . "Is it okay now?" I asked.

"Yep, that was it," Meredith answered.

"I mean, is it, does it *sound* okay?"

"All the facts are there." She hesitated. "It's not your usual—there's nothing—it doesn't sound like *you*. . . . Is that what you mean?"

 That is NOT what I mean. Just yes or no, a simple OK.

"Oh, Suz, I'm sorry, I thought that's what you were asking."

"It's okay." I had to go; I was crying. "Bye." It *had* been what I was asking when she took me to the clinic, but that was Friday, four days ago. *If I keep comparing, reminding myself how I used to sound or be, I'll never feel like doing anything again.*

She was crying when I hung up on her. Neither of us called back. We weren't mad, or I was mad at too many other things to notice. It was too hard. For me: *She* was a reminder of how I used to be. For her: She knew too well how I felt, and for the first time in our lives, she didn't know what to say or do to comfort me. We didn't talk to each other for five weeks.

My therapist hugged me hello and I sat on the couch. Her two cocker spaniels jumped up and sat, one on either side of me. She sat in a rocker facing the three of us, the window above the couch lighting her face. There was a clock above the window that made birdcalls on the hour.

I patted the dogs. I felt some pressure, some obligation—*you're the one who requested the appointment*—to start the conversation. *Each minute is costing $1.66.*

"Well, how's Suzy?" she finally asked.

"You think I need"—*What are they called?*—"pills?"

"Do you?"

"Dr. Finn's doctor did."

"We can talk about it."

I was self-conscious; she was a new audience. I was aware, again, of the strain in my voice, the cramp in my jaw. My tongue felt foreign. It's surprising how quickly you can get used to things.

"You're speaking slow-ly," she over-enunciated.

"Mm. I don't know if I can work again."

"What are they telling you?"

"I'm fine. It will go away. They don't know."

"Don't know?"

"They said twenty-fourth—one day. Now one month. Before, they said my right side. Not this."

"It's too early to tell, isn't it? It's hard not knowing."

MY LIFE LINE

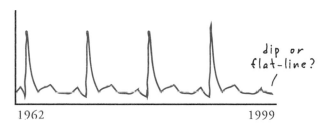

My therapist broke the silence. "I have another client who had brain surgery. She's trying to figure out what's next. It's a lot to cope with, a major shift in your identity, remaking yourself. . . . It's a lot of work, and it's not clear at this point whether you need to do it."

There *had* been times I had considered changing therapists, but this wasn't one of them. How many therapists had a husband *and* a client who'd

---

MEMO

TO: ___Old Therapist___   SUBJECT: ___Baggage___
                                          ___Transfer___

MESSAGE:

Please use the cable enclosed (directions attached) to download any files from your head on to the zip disk (also enclosed) and forward along with any paper files (using the labels provided) to my new therapist. Thank you for your help in the past and in advance for expediting this process.

SIGNED: ___Suzy___

---

had brain surgery? "Think I could talk to her?"

She shook her head. "Not right now. Can't Dr. Finn connect you with someone?"

That was a good idea; I would call him. I thought for a while again. *Here's a positive spin.* "This, this could answer some questions. Maybe about my spirit." I had questions we never answered before when Harriet, my eighty-year-old friend and role model, was succumbing to Alzheimer's. From what I could see, the spirit didn't wait for the body, for the moment of death, to move on. "Um. Who am I? Without my brain?" *Maybe, without my brain in control, my spirit might step up, take over. . . .* "And, I want to paint."

"Oh, yeah? You've been saying that for a long time."

"I am—going to buy an easel. I'm scared about money."

"Don't make this harder on yourself." She never gave advice outright, like that. "That's why you have savings."

"I don't know what to do—the Bunting."

"You don't need a fellowship to—" When she said that, I started crying. "It's too early."

"I have—papers due—"

"Already?"

> "If I am not the same," wondered Alice, "the next question is, who in the world am I? Ah, that's the great puzzle!"
>
> —LEWIS CARROLL,
> *ALICE IN WONDERLAND*

Not term papers. "Paperworks—forms. And, I don't know if I can do Ride FAR."

"The biking?"

"The rest."

"Can you let it go for a couple of weeks?"

"He said onth—one month. He said to go on vacation."

"Why don't you?"

"I have testing tomorrow." That was an upsetting thought. I was quiet.

"Where are you?" she asked.

"Testing. It's so bad." There was the birdcall; a full hour had gone by.

"Why are they throwing you into it so soon? You don't have to—"

I didn't let her finish. "I want to get better."

She reached for her appointment book. "Is next Tuesday good?"

She wrote the appointment on the back of her business card and handed it to me. "Scary times, huh?" She hugged me again.

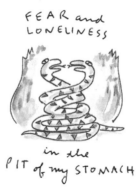

FEAR and LONELINESS

in the PIT of my STOMACH

I'd been home only a few minutes when Stan wheeled his lawn mower up. "I thought you might have an easier time with this." He pushed a button, and it started right up. We both stood there, staring at it running; then he killed the motor.

"Thanks, Stan."

"No problem." He looked down at the mower, then back up at me. "Margaret and I were saying we wished you'd let us know. We would've liked to help out. We don't feel like very good neighbors, that's all."

"It was fast—happened fast, Stan."

"But you're going to be okay?"

"Think so."

"You know Arthur"—Stan looked across the street at Arthur's house—"has been fighting some cancer. He was getting treatments over the winter. We didn't find out until the spring."

First I'd heard of it. Now I felt like a bad neighbor.

"He seems okay," Stan added. "He's back working and everything. . . . Well, call me when you're done, and I'll come pick it up. I could do it for you . . ." It wasn't an afterthought, more of a foregone rejection.

I traded my black hat for a blue baseball cap, opened to the largest size so it could sit on my head. It took an hour to finish the lawn. Then I refilled the gas tank and wheeled it back to Stan's. (It was much easier than calling.) No one was home, so I left it in front of the garage and made a mental note to keep an eye on it in case of rain.

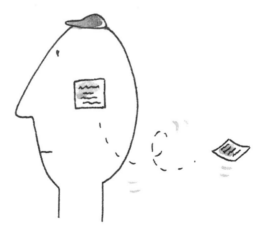

Karen took me to Mister's vet appointment. The three of us went in to the animal hospital. The vet examined Mister's eye. It was time to take the next step. "Basically, you have three options . . ." At first I was following what he was saying.

Then I wasn't. I took my eyes off the vet to make sure Karen was following as he was just finishing up. He and Karen were looking at me.

The Options and the Table

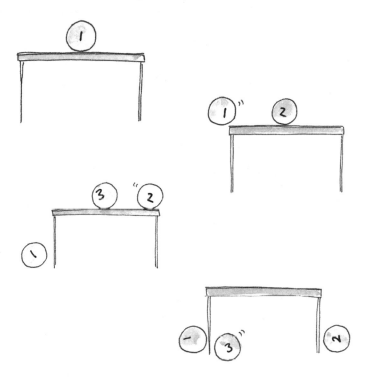

"What do you think, Suz?"

I think I can forget about having a baby, since I can't even take care of a dog. "Nn. Not sure. You?"

"Makes sense to do what he says."

Which?

"Then you'll need to drop him off on Friday. No food or water after midnight," the vet said.

I'd just agreed to surgery.

I waited until we were in the car. "I didn't understand."

"Which part?"

"Any. Tues— Christ! Friday—what's Friday?"

"He's going to put Mister out so he can really take a good look at the eye. Then he's going to stitch it shut so nothing gets in, which'll give it a chance to heal. It was either that or wait six weeks to see a specialist, who would then put him out to look at the eye—or, he said you could do nothing, live with it, although that could permanently damage the cornea. Even waiting six weeks for the specialist . . ."

Mister had never been under anesthesia before. I felt a headache lurking at the edges of my brain. *Let it be.* I trusted the vet the way I trusted Dr. Finn.

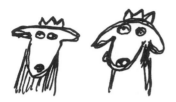

please whatever's watching out
for my brain I know I'm not
the most grateful - please also
look out Mister's eye.

By the time we got to Somerville, Karen was dizzy from exhaustion, and her jaw was aching. It was her turn to be the princess. I tried to take care of her. *I don't have what it takes.* We both sank into bed in an inconsolable state.

What It Takes
humor
patience
thick skin
generosity
not being tired

ALL the TEA in CHINA

Behavioral observation: During the second testing session she
seemed less frustrated and less discouraged.

Wrong. I was just more prepared to suffer the humiliation. And seeing how I never so much as laid eyes on Deborah Knight (her assistant administered all the testing), she had no grounds for comparison.

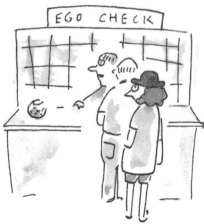

The assistant was casually dressed, a Harvard grad student in her late twenties. She was nice and patient and, I wanted to believe, empathetic.

She got out the fat notebook again; this time there were two pictures, side by side. I was to identify what they had in common.

"Transportation."

I knew most of the pairs, or knew I used to know, until this one:

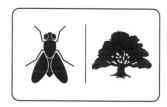

The scale was distracting. I couldn't think of anything, and the longer I tried, the less I could think. "Both outside." She didn't respond. "Same ecosystem." *Same shit, more syllables.*

"Can you say more about that?"

I pretended to think before answering no.

"What *is* the answer?"

"I'm sorry—I can't tell you."

The picture pairs were followed by more word problems. I took turns telling myself: *I could have answered that if it was written down* and *That has no relevance to my work.*

Next she handed me a piece of paper. "We're going to draw.

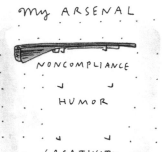

my ARSENAL

NONCOMPLIANCE

HUMOR

CREATIVITY

Fun. Where's YOUR paper?

There is a design on the paper I am about to hand you. I want you to copy this design, exactly as you see it, onto the blank piece of paper you have in front of you."

I looked at the geometric design, and I felt a rush of confidence, an alertness I hadn't felt since the surgery. I moved the blank piece closer. *Draw what you see. Break it down into smaller shapes.* I coached myself the way I'd coached kids.

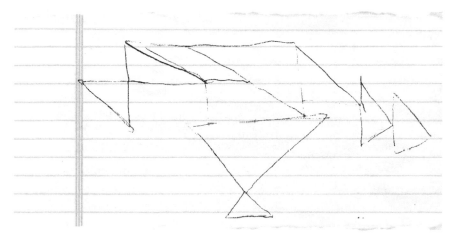

A little juvenile. A mild motor deficit, but not bad overall. I was pleased with my work.

She took the paper (no feedback) and handed me another blank sheet. *Straight lines have always been a relative weakness—ask me to draw a rabbit, a car, anything—bring it on!*

"Now I'd like you to draw the same figure from memory. You may begin."

So this was the *real* test. I swallowed, trying to press the queasiness back down. She sat there, tabulating my results; the pencil-scritching was making static of my memory.

"If I just put shapes, not—?" I asked.

She looked up. "Sorry, I can't help you with this one."

Degree of QUEASINESS

 Sorry, I forgot to thank you for all your help on the other ones.

I stared at the blank paper until she said, "Time!" I lifted my arms so she could take the paper away.

There were at least four more tests: math, logic, reasoning, and planning, and then, the last, a long written test of my ability to organize information. She left the room while I took it. I had just finished when she popped her head in. "Five minutes!"

"I'm done." I meant to let her know, but the tone of my voice (which I couldn't control) sounded defiant.

"Why don't you use the extra time to check your work?"

"I'm done—thanks."

Karen was in the waiting area. She put her arms around me, waiting for me to go limp, then ventured, "Was it okay?"

"What's the same—how are a tree and a fly the same?"

She thought for a minute. "I don't know." That was all I felt like saying. "Shall we go get an easel?"

What's the point? It's not just my words—everything is ruined. I am not interested in art therapy—making pictures like Harriet's. The nurses in the dementia ward hung them on the wall as if she hadn't had a show at a gallery just the year before.

We stood, surrounded by easels, in the basement of the art supply store. "I don't know how to pick."

"Neither do I. Ask for help."

I *was* asking. I wanted to leave.

"I'd like an easel." The clerk had plugs in his earlobes four times the size of my mother's hearing aids. I touched my ear reflexively and added, "The best value." I took the first one he pointed to and let him carry the box up to the register. Karen was still browsing. I walked up to the second floor to pick out some oil sticks: Naples yellow, pale gray.

From time to time, there were beautiful, peculiar images in my head. I wasn't sure if they were my own or somebody else's—Chagall's maybe, in a palette of yellows, grays, pale and deep blues. They flickered, then faded, like dreams. I tried to remember the details, but all that was left was a swatch of color: yellow, red, or vivid blue.

None of the blues were perfect; but I chose two: azure and turquoise. I was reaching for gold, craving shinyness, then reconsidered. Opalescent white.

That night, Karen and I went to see *The Buena Vista Social Club*. I was awash in color again, and music. No words. *Maybe I should go to Cuba on vacation.* Karen squeezed my hand. *Maybe she'd come with me.* She pulled my arm hard, and I looked over.

"Let's go," she said, and started to stand. "C'mon, let's just go." I craned my head around to see if I had missed something. "I'm sorry, sweetie; I didn't know about the subtitles."

I pulled her back down. "No." The people on all four sides shifted. She was trying to see my eyes. "I'm okay."

I couldn't get back into the movie. The subtitles, which I hadn't noticed before, blinked noisily across the bottom of the screen. *How can she be sitting so close and think I was hating it?*

The movie let out. I waited for Karen to say something on the walk home. Finally, she said, "I don't think I'm the best person for you, Suz. . . . Your lover should be your best friend."

We've had this conversation before; it's actually an argument that I never win, even when the playing field is level.

"Your lover is your lover," I said.

"No one *has* been a better friend through all this than I've been."

I don't know. She was looking for reassurance. *No one's been a better— something. Bruce doesn't need reassurance, but then again Bruce hasn't been taking care of me. I don't know.* I didn't answer.

I QUIT!

We had said good night, and Karen had rolled over, but I knew she was awake. Her hand twitches when she falls off to sleep.

I stared at her back. "Maybe you could go to Maine."

"Everything's here. All my books."

"Maybe you should see your friends."

"Suz, I'm not *like* you. I don't need to surround myself with a lot of people. I don't want to see anyone. That's work for me. I just want to be with you."

I work alone. That's work for me, was work. Now seeing people is work, too. You were so afraid of losing me. Can't you see? I'm lost.

She wasn't afraid of losing me, she just didn't want me to die.

I just want to rest.

Neither of us slept much. I stayed in bed the next morning, where I felt the most out of her way. *What I want, what I really want, what I would trade all the pillows, all the reminders, all the advice, be carefuls, teas in China, right arms and eyeteeth for is someone (Karen) to lie down next to me, hold me, and feel scared with me. As scared as I am that I can't speak, read, or write the way I used to, might never again. To talk about how it feels, what it means.* I fantasized about the relief, the respite from the loneliness, just for maybe fifteen minutes in bed.

THe DANGER

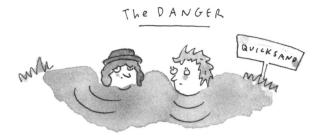

My friend Amy came to take Mister and me to the quarries by her house on the north shore. Once we were on the highway—radio on, windows open—I practiced reading signs, seeing if I could say them under my breath before we passed them. I wasn't much of a driving companion. Amy didn't seem to care.

We stopped to pick up a sandwich not far from her house. The deli had every possible kind of meat, cheese, and condiment and six kinds of bread. My old self always knew exactly what I wanted. I tried to clear a space in my head for some hunch or hunger, a taste or a picture to appear.

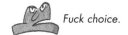 *Fuck choice.*

"Amy, what's good?"

"Everything."

Of course. She ordered. I ordered, "Chicken soup." Only one kind of soup to choose from in July, and my stomach found the idea settling. I paid for both lunches. "You gave her a twenty?" I nodded. Amy turned back to the register. "She gave you a twenty." Now that she'd said it, I doubted myself. *Maybe it was a ten.*

The cashier clunked her forehead with the palm of her hand. "I thought that wasn't right." She handed Amy a ten and apologized.

After lunch, we walked the dogs through the woods to the quarries. Granite slabs, cleaved open, the crevices filled with pools of clear water. We spread out towels and lay down on a rock. The dogs swam and shook and sniffed. They found an old tennis ball and dropped it with a soggy thud next to one of us, or more insistently, on a stomach. *Throw!* Amy talked. Her partner was finishing school; she wanted to open a business. It was going to be a big transition for them.

It was my turn. *I have an identity problem—crisis? No. I'm trying to get my self back, get back to myself.* The words would come crashing back down, flattening us on the rocks. I didn't say anything, kept my eyes closed. I wondered if I'd ever recover the empathy, the patience to listen to

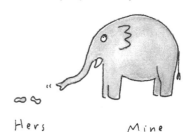

everyday problems—the comparatively small complaints, glitches, inconveniences—the things that people talk about. If I'd forget their smallness and talk about them, too. . . .

I must have fallen asleep. I woke up feeling baked, lying on my back, no familiar ceiling above; I turned my head to orient myself. Amy's towel was empty. I sat up. She was at the water's edge. "Wanna swim, Suz?"

It would feel good to rinse off the film of sleep and sweat. I stood up.

"Careful, it's deep here," Amy warned. "The rocks just drop off."

"How deep?" *I sound like a nonswimmer.* I'd known how to swim for as long as I'd known how to read. I peered down into the black water; it was possible I'd forgotten. I wish I'd thought of that before I stood up—it would have been easier to beg off. Easier to test the waters at home, alone, wading in Little Pond, Bolton's beach, with a sandy bottom half a leg's length below.

The dogs were standing on the rocks, watching. "You okay, Suz?" Amy adjusted her suit, getting ready to go in.

"Fine." I said. "Go." She dived. I winced when her head broke the water. I'd have to jump. Away from the rock, but close enough to grab on, just in case. *One, two, three. One, two, okay. One, two—* I threw my arms up and plunged.

I didn't fight the water on my way down, through the light into the dark. *Still no bottom in sight.* I brought my arms down to my sides and kicked back up through the light water and into the air. I rolled over, floated on my back, on my stomach, and took a few breaststrokes with my head out of the water. Then I put my face down and kicked, turning my arms, windmills. Breathed right, breathed left, plunged my right arm deeper, diving down, turning, ending up on my back again. It was all there! The sky, the sun, the shore, the dogs . . .

Mister saw me surface and did a running dive. We hadn't been swimming since he was a pup, last August; then he'd clung to me like a toddler, front paws on my shoulders, back legs still paddling. At sixty-five pounds, in my weakened state, he could pull me under.

"Should I call him, Suz?" Amy swam toward me.

"I'm okay." She kept a stick to throw at the ready. *I think he knows.* Mister hadn't jumped up at or stepped on my head in the seven days I'd been home—the longest I'd gone without a cut or bruise on my face since I got him.

He was within an arm's length. I reached out and smoothed his ears, and he came about. I roughed his neck and followed him in to shore, retrieved. He stood dripping wet, looking pleased while I pulled myself out; then he went over to shake off by Amy.

Amy drove me home. My mother was bringing another picnic; this time she was staying. She and Karen would be waiting for me. I rested my head on the seat. I could still feel the sun, rock, water—and now the air, all four windows open, washing over me.

I couldn't wait to see Karen.

I think I feel better today — maybe my
medication tapering.
And for the first time writing Lorene ı Randi
I felt like I had my sense of humor back.
I thought it would feel better to write in here.
disappointingly slow, belabored at usual.
I'm going to set up my easel tomorrow.

BEE'S-EYE VIEW

Karen was waiting in my studio when I got home from dropping Mister off for his eye surgery. They'd had to drag him—he never stopped looking at me—into the back. "It was hard." I started crying. I was so sick of crying. I hated myself this way. *The new me.*

Karen put her glasses on. "Where's your Bunting stuff, sweetie?" I handed her the envelope with all the paperwork. The colloquium sign-up sheet was on top. "What's your project title?"

"Don't know."

"Haven't you been calling it *Fertile Mind?*"

I can't call it that. "It has to sell the coll-l."

colloquium: an academic seminar usually led by a different lecturer at each meeting

"It's Harvard—I don't think you have to worry about selling." I didn't say anything. "Suz, when are you going to tell them?"

I don't know. I wish I'd told them before. My jig was up. I couldn't even make a phone call, let alone a colloquium. "Monday. As long as Mister is okay." *Don't you think I've had enough stress for one day?*

"It's summer, it's a university—on a Friday—no one's going to be there. It'll take two seconds to leave a message."

What would I say? I didn't want anyone calling me back when I wasn't prepared to have a conversation. *An intellectually rigorous conversation.*

"Let's practice."

"You do it. How will they know?"

She wagged her finger at me.

"Hi—" *Christ.* I couldn't remember how a message went.

"Hi, this is Suzy Becker," Karen prompted. "It's not like you want to say 'I had brain surgery' in the message— Hi, this is Suzy Becker, and I was just filling in the questionnaire— FLAG! Three syllables! Okay, I was—"

"Please. Can't *you* just?"

"Hi, Renny, this is Suzy Becker. When you get a chance, please give me a call. I'm at— 978-779-0401." Karen's eyebrows arched; my turn.

The number was going to be the hardest part. I wrote the whole message out and read it aloud to Karen, three times. Then she dialed the number, handed me the phone, and went downstairs.

"Hi, this is Renny." *OHMYGOD! I have to hang up.*

"Nn hi Renny—this is Suzy Becker." Karen crept back upstairs.

"Suzy Becker, how are you? What can I do for you?"

"That's why I'm calling"—*What's why, you idiot?*—"I had surgery— on my brain?" My nervous laugh formed a question mark.

"My god, Suzy. That's some news. Are you okay?"

"Think I will be—in a month. It shcrew—messed up my shpeech." *Screwed? Screwed? Jesus, Suzy.*

"Well, the brain has remarkable healing powers. My son had meningitis when he was very young; he had to relearn all kinds of things, motor things. . . . Is there anything we can do for you?" She paused. "I wish you'd let me know, we would've sent you something. When was the operation?"

"June. Sept"—*Goddamn*—"July fourth, I mean second." *I sound like a pathological liar with Tourette's.* It was worse when I was nervous.

"Two weeks ago? Sounds like you're doing very well. Listen, if you need to start late, that's not a problem."

"I'm not sure about the coll-colll—"

"We can cross that bridge when we come to it—what's the worst? We cancel it—no big deal. You worry about getting better."

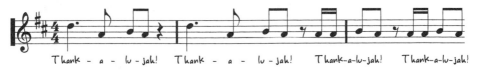

Thank - a - lu - jah! Thank - a - lu - jah! Thank-a-lu-jah! Thank-a-lu-jah!

"You know, I wanted to tell you"—*I thought we were done*—"your writing sample, that macrobiotic piece, is the funniest thing I've read in a long time! My son spent some time at that place you wrote about. . . .

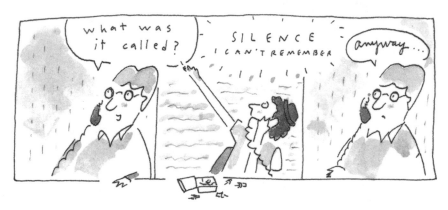

"It's all so serious. I guess that's what makes it funny, right?"

"Mm."

"I just wanted to say congratulations."

"Thanks, Renny. Thank you for picking me." *I hope you won't regret it.*

Mister was no longer sedated when we went to pick him up, not the slightest bit subdued. He looked pitiful, lurching down the hall toward us with his head in a plastic cone. The sewn-shut eye was quivering. *Does it try to open every time he blinks?* I pressed my eyelid closed and blinked; I could feel the eyeball moving, but I couldn't tell if—Karen nudged me. The receptionist had finished going over the discharge instructions and was asking for my credit card. "When did you want to schedule the recheck?" She flipped the pages of her oversize appointment calendar noisily. "How's the thirtieth?"

"Mm."

I should be able to fit that in . . .

That night, Mister pulled out of his cone going up the stairs to Karen's. Karen stepped over the cone to let Molly in; she was at the sink filling the dogs' water bowl *forever.*

FEDERAL EMERGENCY!

"Help!" I yelled from the hallway. *He's going to scratch his eye out!* I picked up the cone.

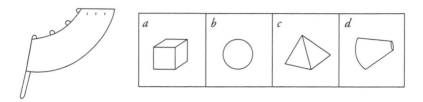

I was starting to hyperventilate. Karen took the cone out of my hands and inspected it. *"Hurry!"* She rolled her eyes. "Then give it back!" She handed it back. "Watch Mister!" My hands were shaking as I tried to put it back together. "Shit!"

She took it from me. "Do you remember what size it was?"

"There aren't sizes."

 You complicate everything!

She showed me the sizes. "But, since you don't remember there were sizes, maybe it went this way."

If your voice gets any calmer I'm going to SCREAM!

She had it. *She's a genius. I love her so much.* I was breathing normally again.

I went to hug her, and she stepped away. "A little kindness couldn't hurt, Suz."

"You don't get it!" I was crying again. "How it is. It's not a choice."

I panicked about Mrs collar coming off last night.

I have to trust I won't end up a mean person who never says thank you *just* because I don't feel like saying it now.

The next day, the temperature had risen back up to a hundred degrees for the fifty-mile training ride. Seven riders, the mechanic, and the head of the road crew were assembled in the parking lot at 9 A.M., awaiting my announcements. I stood in front of them, holding a stack of papers, not in bike shorts, but everyone was too absorbed in their own preparations to notice.

"Couple of things." I cleared my throat, trying to dislodge my voice. "I'm not riding." All eyes were on me. "Today." (Throat.) "I had brain surgery." All eyes shifted to my baseball cap. "I'll be okay. Just need to rest today." I continued with the announcements; my tongue got irretrievably tied on the times and dates of the upcoming events, at which point I passed out a calendar. They could read for themselves. "Laura is me, today." She'd be riding last, sweep.

"Tammy and I decided on the way over," Laura said, "that we're going to do twenty-five miles. I, for one, don't feel like riding fifty miles in the middle of a hundred-degree day."

Well, thanks for sharing that with me beforehand.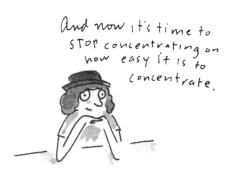

The others all nodded in agreement. I'd been usurped.

I tried to help a rider pump her tire and then retired to the sidelines. *Am I just being controlling? What if it's one hundred degrees on the ride? Would the old me have made the same call?* The troubling part was, I didn't know.

ICP
ALERT!

I went home and drafted a letter to the rest of the Ride FAR participants. I was glad I'd left myself a clean office, an empty white desk, to start out with. It was easier to concentrate.

And now it's time to STOP concentrating on how easy it is to concentrate.

The phone rang; I didn't pick up. It was Laura; everyone had safely finished the training ride and was on their way home. *Maybe I'll write the letter on Monday.* I glanced at the calendar. *Six days until I can get back on my bike.*

The phone rang again, and this time, without thinking, I picked up. "Hi, darlin'! How are you!" It was Jim, a California rider. Six foot six, movie-star looks, year-round tan. "Everything must be coming together for the ride—you must be going kind of crazy! Honey, I'm doing my damnedest to ride this thing! My doc can't get a handle on this prostate cancer. I've been so-o-o sick." He never sounded sick. And he never complained. Last time we talked, his T-cell count was under ten.

"It's still a few weeks, Jim. . . . We have the van." Such meager words.

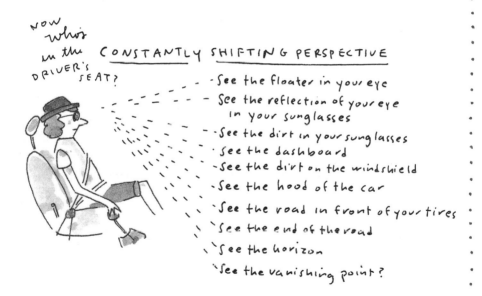

NOW who's in the DRIVER's SEAT?

CONSTANTLY SHIFTING PERSPECTIVE

- See the floater in your eye
- See the reflection of your eye in your sunglasses
- See the dirt in your sunglasses
- See the dashboard
- See the dirt on the windshield
- See the hood of the car
- See the road in front of your tires
- See the end of the road
- See the horizon
- See the vanishing point?

I was twenty-five minutes late for my Tuesday therapist appointment. "I got lost," I said before I sat down, one of those excuses that was so hard to believe, it had to be true.

She didn't seem perturbed. "Have you come up with any answers?"

"To?"

"Last week, we ended with your question, 'Who am I without my brain?'"

That was *last* week. This week, it seemed more constructive to identify all my missing parts, and then make a plan to recover them.

"What's missing?" she asked.

"Things I was tested on . . . Whistling. I don't know—yet, all the things. I have to find out."

"How are you going to do that?"

I didn't know that either; it was a new plan. Up until now, I didn't know things were missing until I went looking for them. I'd have to speed up that process, devote more time to it. *What about the things I don't think to look for?*

"Why didn't they do any neuropsych testing before the surgery?"

"It was just my right side—not my shpeech." It was some annoying ironic stupid joke, the way I could never say *speech.*

"What would it feel like to feel like 'yourself' again? Have you thought about that?"

"Independent." I couldn't come up with *autonomous.* "Not afraid." I wanted to say *alive,* but it sounded too dramatic. I didn't know how else to describe the feeling, that current I used to feel. "Feel the urge to make things. Love people. Oh, to make people laugh." *I used to live for that. Now what do I live for?*

"To be thoroughly engaged?" She was parroting my old words back at me. They sounded so far out or up there, I wanted to laugh almost as much as I wanted to cry.

"To feel big—to not feel so small."

"Have you thought about the antidepressants?" *She thinks I need them.*

"No—I don't think it's, I mean *I'm* wrong. It *is* depressing."

"The medication can take away some of the anxiety, maybe help you feel more like yourself."

"I think I'm getting better. I feel better. This is my first day off all the pills. Except Neurontin." *This would be where you say you think I'm getting better, too.*

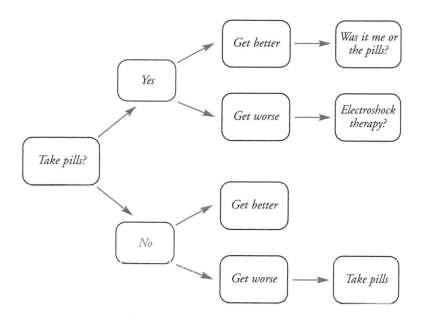

"I'm not a pill person. They make some people feel better. They make me feel . . . like a sick person." *You could at least nod.* "Um. I wish I had some steps"—*not steps, what do you call them?*—"word like *goals?*"

"Milestones? Benchmarks?" *Right.* "Did Dr. Finn's office have someone for you to—?"

"They're calling me back."

"What about a vacation?"

"I wanted to wait until my tests came back."

"How were they?"

I shrugged, made a face under my hat.

"Are you painting?"

"The easel is set up."

"Resting?"

"Then I'm not tired at night."

"Why don't you listen to music?"

I had that box of CDs from Darleen and Alan. . . . I turned to look at the clock. Five of. "Next Thursday?"

"Would Thursday work better?"

Christ. "I meant Today"—*not today!*—"Tood-Tues-day."

Dr. Finn's office called back. There wasn't anyone they felt comfortable suggesting. Nobody's experience really resembled mine, and Dr. Finn didn't want me forming expectations based on somebody else's experience. "We'll just have to wait and see," the nurse said. "We'll know more on the thirtieth!" *Ten more days of wait and see.*

What if I promise not to form any expectations? What if I just want to talk to someone who's been through this—I remembered the aneurysm story my neighbor had told me and called her. She said she'd have to double-check with her friend and get back to me. Less than ten minutes later, she called back. "She said you could call. She's in her office now."

Instant nervous stomach.

NEVER CALL	POSTPONE CALL	CALL NOW
+ never nervous	+ not nervous now	+ comfort now?
− never comforted	− postpone comfort	− nervous

You're not asking her for a job or a date—just call.

"Alyson Caldwell."

It took me a second. *Why doesn't anyone have receptionists anymore?* "Hi. This is a friend of Cathy Freed's. Suzy Becker."

"I'm really glad you called. Let me close my door." I held. "How many weeks has it been?"

"Three. Two. Sorry, my numbers. I had surgery on July two. Second."

"You sound good. You sound better than I did, I think, although my speech came back pretty quickly. I had more trouble with reading and writing, I guess, and thinking. Concentration was a big problem." *Yes!* "But, it took me a long time before I could admit I had a problem. I waited six months before I was tested."

"Six months off?"

"Oh, no, I went back to work after—I can't remember whether it was three or four weeks—and basically hid. I'm an editor. I would go to meetings and not say much. Hide in my office." *Oh, I wish I had a job where I could hide.* "I worried that people would find out. I had one friend I could talk to; I would go into her office, and she would reassure me whatever I was feeling wasn't noticeable to anybody else. Maybe, she said, I was a little quieter, but that was all. I guess that was how I was able to face it finally, realizing nobody else was going to call me on it. It was my problem."

"I've already been tested."

"Well, see, you're ahead of the game. Do you have your results?"

"Some."

"After six months, my reading comprehension was in the sixtieth percentile for a college graduate. Now I think it's above where it was before the surgery. I'm definitely a much better worker as a result of all this. I learned things in therapy I'd never really been taught before. I'm a much more organized person, and my concentration—I'm able to focus for much longer."

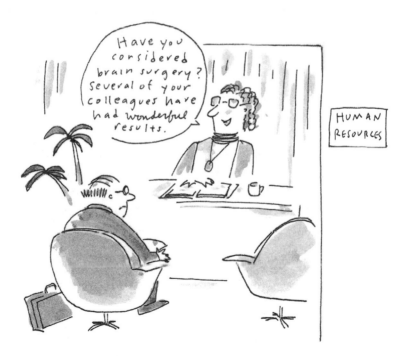

"I'm afraid they can't help me. I'm a writer and an artist."

"You have to be kind of pushy. Adamant. It's not about what *they* think is okay, or what's okay for some truck driver or even what's okay for me—it's what's okay for you. This *is* Boston, not—I don't know—Iowa or something. I'm sure they've worked with artists before . . . but, don't worry about it until the time comes. Enjoy your time off. I don't know what it's like for you—I was single at the time, and I remember having a bunch of chairs set up in my yard, and my mother and friends would come over—"

"Could you talk? I mean, converse, conversation?"

"Oh, no. No, no, I let other people talk. Sometimes I would listen. Sometimes I would sleep and someone would tuck a towel or blanket around me."

It sounded idyllic. *What's wrong with me, why don't I just relax? What people would give for a few weeks off in the summer . . .* "Um. Did you have a sense of humor?"

"I don't know. All I remember was I was pretty out of it those first few weeks—listen—" She was going to end the call.

"Weren't you ever scared you'd never be yourself again?" I had to ask.

"God, yes. I didn't mean to make it sound like, well, what have I made it sound like?"

"I'm sorry—" Her "God, yes" was such a relief I was crying. "People keep saying you, I sound fine. Like this is a vacation." I didn't mean her.

"I'm sorry. Suzy, I'll tell you what got me through: denial. A lot of denial. So you screw things up. You can't do something you used to be able to do. Ignore it. I'm totally serious. People say you sound fine, you're the only one who notices—notice the things you do right. Let the rest go."

I can't let them go or they're gone—don't you see? If I'm the only one who notices—who's going to get them back?

That afternoon, I actually had some place to go besides, or in addition to, the doctor's. (My pelvic ultrasound was at 7 P.M.) My friend Carol and I were going to the John Singer Sargent show at the Museum of Fine Arts.

The show was packed. The paintings were huge. The captions were tiny. I found myself more interested in looking at the people than at the art; then, paranoid I was missing something, I'd turn to look at what they were looking at. I finally came to a grouping of watercolors at the end that held my attention. They were small, more loosely drawn, and lightly painted. I peered through the paint at the paper beyond.

Carol tapped my shoulder. "I love this show. Did you read—?" She stopped as if she'd brought up someone who'd just died.

"The words shouldn't be so small. Or white on"— *What do you call that color?*—"dark red."

DENIAL

I left Carol at the museum shop. I had to get home in time to drink thirty-two ounces of water before going to the ultrasound. I pulled into the driveway at six of six, which was six minutes under the bathroom deadline. I raced to the door; Mister was waiting for me on the other side. The inside of his cone was coated with black powder. A mystery. A *dog* mystery, which meant there had to be clues. I was heading for his couch when I remembered his eyes— *Black powder is getting in his eyes!* I had to get the cone off— Then I saw the mess. He'd emptied a canister of graphite powder all over the cushions, throw pillows, rug. I grabbed the pillows— *No, first his eyes. Oh, god, the fluids, shit, the bathroom—too late! Stop. Stop crying. Get ahold of yourself.*

I measured the fluids and gulped down the thirty-two ounces straight out of the measuring cup.

Next, his eyes. I had to wash the cone. I ran the water. *I can't take it off; he'll scratch his eyes. Where's Robin? Goddamn water is making me have to go to the bathroom.* I sponged the cone. Black water ran toward his eyes. I tried to towel the inside out. *Then keep the towel, you little shit.* While Mister held on to the towel, I pulled the cone over his head, washed it, dried it, and dragged his head back through. Still no Robin. *Maybe I should go alone. You find out you have cancer alone, you die alone. Really, what's the difference?*

My vacuum cleaner, which can supposedly suck up an eight-pound bowling ball, made black graphite powder clouds in the den. I turned it off, grabbed the pillows, and stepped outside the kitchen door to bang them together. More clouds.

A BEE'S-EYE VIEW

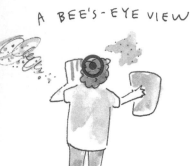

I ran inside, then outside, swinging the pillow wildly, bees on my trail—then I let the pillows fly (with most of the bees following) and ran back inside. I was lying on the kitchen floor, sobbing, *I can't take it anymore* . . . when Robin arrived. Mister gave up trying to get his cone over my face and went to lick Robin instead.

"I'm okay," I sobbed. She knelt and hugged me. "We have—have to go." She was silent. The next day she said it scared her, seeing me lose it like that.

By the time I lay down on the ultrasound table, I have never had to go the bathroom more fiercely in my entire life. I watched the technician's face. "Normal. Beautiful, in fact. Look." She turned the monitor toward us.

I rehearsed the sentence in my head. "The last woman said I could be a model."

"You could. Definitely!"

She swiveled the monitor back. "All done!"

My relief was profound.

Im ~~beginning~~ (Jinx) to feel like I might be normal again.

COMING THROUGH!

My agent called in the morning. The contract finally came through for the I Can Read book. "What if I can't write it?" I asked.

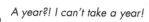

How 'bout an I Can'T Read book?

"Don't worry—we won't actually see the contract for another three weeks, and the book's not due until March or April."

"Don't tell him about my—"

"Of course not. There's no need to. April is a long way off. . . . A friend of ours had brain surgery, a medical doctor. He ended up taking a year off.

A year?! I can't take a year!

"After a year, he had recovered ninety percent of"—she hesitated—"of himself. He's been able to resume his practice."

The story was reassuring, in a way; I was going to need more than a month to get better. (It had been almost three weeks, and the pace of my recovery had slowed substantially since the first week.) It was the 90 percent part—*I know it's only minus 10 percent, but . . .* I didn't want to go through my life feeling less than 100 percent, less than who I used to be.

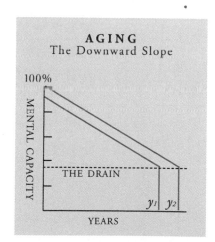

I sat and drafted my Ride FAR fund-raising letter at my desk. After rewriting the original several times—my hand (like my mouth) had developed a mind of its own—I resorted to liberal applications of white-out.

RIDE FAR 6

NEXT TIME I'LL TRY A GIMMICK...

This time I'm too far behind, and besides, I'm supposed to be resting. I had brain surgery (just some scar tissue that didn't even qualify as a tumor) on the 2nd of July. I watched the fireworks over the Esplanade from the 16th floor of the hospital and then I got outta there the 5th.

The doctors say my concentration will improve over the next month but in the meantime . . .

HERE'S MY POINT: With more help than ever, I am organizing Ride FAR 6, the sixth 5-day 500-mile fund-raising bike-a-thon for children and adults with AIDS. The first five have raised over $275,000 and all of that money has gone directly to AIDS service organizations. (None has gone to administration, production, or hats.)

In going ahead with the ride, riders and road crew decided to forgo some of the donations that make the ride more comfortable (not safe), in order to concentrate on raising the most funds possible. I hope you'll support my commitment to reaching our goal. And now where was I ~~doing the dishes,~~ ~~watering~~, resting.

See ya, Suzy

I mailed the first batch on my way to the HIV Treatment Update meeting that Ride FAR sponsors. I was supposed to say a few words—nothing major, just a couple of sentences from my seat when I was introduced by the local AIDS project director.

The director, it turned out, also had a stuttering problem. I borrowed his line ("easy for *me* to say") when I attempted my sentence about the Ride FAR benefit concert for the third time. I'd rehearsed this particular sentence over and over, so my brain had all the phrases on-line; it just shot them out in random order—the ticket price in place of the date, the time in place of the ticket price. Take four: "I have a flyer! Thanks y—thank you all for coming." I half stood, half sat while they applauded politely.

Mike, a veteran Ride FAR rider, and I went out for pie afterwards. "Becks," he said, "they were in there a coupla weeks ago messing with your brain, and you just stood up in there—"

His acknowledgment made me feel self-conscious again. "I'm getting better." My difficulties seemed so abstract, so superficial after this meeting, where people's alarms and beepers kept going off to remind them to down a handful of pills. "I don't know about working. I used to hear voices, characters in my head. It's empty now. Speaking is so hard, they all quit—I don't know."

 Mail Message

Becks,
I'm imagining the "voices" you mentioned over key lime pie on Wednesday, and how they seem to you to be temporarily AWOL. . . . Here's the deal as I see it. . . . They are very much safe and sound in some other part of your head, waiting for the All Clear Signal, as in "Are you completely through, Doc, with the noise from the itty-bitty saw and the bright lights and the freakin' metal toys and all the rest?" And I'm figuring a nice, safe place to hang out for a while is behind the junk you learned in high school about plane geometry and in among that very complex and most important part: exactly how you go about hoisting up those exquisite VBall sets that are such works o' art.

L/Mick

Mike, it occurred to me, was an example of what the psychiatrist in Dr. Finn's office had been talking about when he asked me if I had ever dealt with disappointment. When we first met in the early 1980s, Mike was an environmental artist. Then he became an environmental activist. In the mid-'90s, he went back to school to get a degree in environmental law, even though he hates school and never did well at it. (He's dyslexic.) He studied harder than anybody I've ever known, got the degree, and failed the bar. He retook the exam and failed twice more. Then he started his own business designing exhibits for law firms.

I'd never faced that kind of disappointment. In my thirty-six years, I'd never had to persevere in the face of failure. *Maybe I don't have what it takes.*

PROGRESS checkLIST

☑ Started training

☑ Scheduled speech therapy

☑ Had ultrasound

☑ Braver about phone

The next Tuesday, I composed a checklist as I sat on my therapist's couch. Not bad, I thought. For one of *these* weeks.

"How are you doing? How'd it go—? Last week you were talking about mapping out some of the missing pieces. . . ."

"Oh." I'd forgotten about that. Remembering it burst my progress bubble. I had a new strategy: look down and keep going. (It worked biking up hills.) Looking up—seeing how long it is taking you to get where you are going—is discouraging.

"Did you paint?" *Add that to the list.* "How'd it go?"

"It's different." I had painted apricots on a field of blue from a photograph of a fruit stand I took in Paris. "Egg yolks?" was the general reaction. (The easel was opposite the mudroom door.) "I think people are worried I can't draw anymore or something."

"Are *you?*"

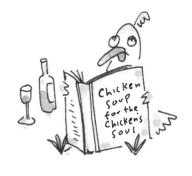

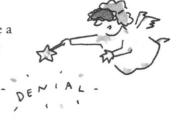

"I don't want to paint now. I don't want to be a beginner. I want to feel good at something. I don't know what I'm good at anymore. . . ." It was kind of a game; everywhere I went I wondered if I could do *that*. "The only job I think I can do is bagging. At the supermarket. I am still good at packing." I laughed, but I wasn't kidding. I had also been considering suicide, although I wasn't suicidal. It opened up my options. If (after some amount of time, TBD) the quality of my life did not meet my minimum standard, I would not force myself to live it. I'd done as much for my dogs.

"Have you heard from your favorite neuropsychologist?"

I was screening calls when she phoned the day before. Her voice, without the red suit, actually sounded friendly, so I picked up. "She gave me the name of a speech—" I couldn't remember the word she used.

"Pathologist?" *Close*. I nodded. "How do you feel about that?"

Like feelings are irrelevant . . . frustrated. "Like I want to start. Anything to get better. He is on vacation."

"Will you fax me a copy of the evaluation?"

"Yep." I should have done it before. I was hiding my high average to superior scores from her; I didn't want her thinking this was anxiety.

"Do you want to talk about antidepressants?"

"Nope." I asked for an appointment in two weeks. Karen and I were thinking about going away—and it was a test: *If she thinks I'm really sick, she'll make me come in one week.*

"Take my number," she said, handing me her card, "just in case."

MENTAL HEALTH

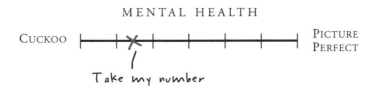

Karen and I decided to go to Ogunquit for a week. Two days before we left, Bruce met me at the bakery for breakfast. It had been a record long time since I'd seen him—four weeks, since the hospital, an unconscious deference to Karen's feelings.

"Want me to ask?" he offered.

"No. I'll ask. *After* breakfast."

"Sure? You might be able to enjoy your breakfast more . . ."

Sure I was sure, except I wasn't hungry. I watched Bruce finish his breakfast, and then I stalled a little longer—the line was too long, the wrong person was at the register—until he said, "I gotta go to work. . . . Think now's a good time?" I nodded. "What do you want me to do?"

"Be there." *In case no words come out.* I stood very close to Bruce at the register. "Hi." The brim of my hat protected me from direct eye contact. "Is there someone I to talk"—*keep going*—"to about my bike-a-thon? A donation to my AIDS ride I organize?" I leaned back into Bruce. *Help.*

The cashier went to get the owner. She came out of the kitchen, wiping her hands on her apron. While I was still in the hospital, I'd thought about getting a job at this bakery, making bread during my convalescence. Soothing work. Nice people. Until I tried baking at home . . .

I handed her a Ride FAR brochure and introduced myself. Then I launched into a solicitation, which after five rides, I knew as well as my own address. The first glitch, "five-day fifty—no, fifteen-hundred, no" derailed the rest of my spiel. "We start and end here in Concord." The End.

Bruce hurriedly tacked on a couple of sentences describing the ride, then looked at me as if I could take it from there. "Do you think you could do the last dinner?"

Bruce again, "Everything is donated; all the money that we raise goes directly to the AIDS service organizations. Nothing to administration . . ." I was grateful he was there, except the part of me that wished nobody had seen any of this.

"I'll have to ask my partners. When do you need to know?" She paused, then answered herself. "I'll let you know in a week."

I waited until we were in the parking lot before I lost it. Bruce ground the sand left over from last winter into the blacktop. "At least it wasn't no," I said. "Maybe I can write a letter, put in everything I left out."

"You can e-mail it to me if you want." I was making him late for work. I walked him to his car, then got in mine and drove home. *If I go up to my desk right away, I'll have four hours.* (I had to be at the Brain Tumor Clinic at two.) *I can write a letter in four hours.*

The first paragraph: why I was writing . . . Skip to the second paragraph: a description of the ride. My stomach balled up. *Why am I putting myself through all this—as if a letter can undo the damage. Wait, use something from an old letter—* The phone rang.

"Suzy, John Gates at the bakery. Karen just showed us the flyer and we are *in!* This is exactly the kind of thing we love to do. We're not usually open on Sunday nights, but my wife will open, cook, take care of everything for you guys. Tell me what you need."

"Thank you, John!" *I can't believe it!* "I was just writing you a letter— I had such a hard time there—" *Wait, let me explain.* "I had brain surgery July second. My shpeech"—*like clockwork—* "is bad."

"You riding this thing?"

"Hope to. Plan to." I was embarrassed I'd said all that. "Sorry."

"I think it's great! I love the graphics—what do you do?"

"Write books and art."

"Would I know any of your books?"

"I'll send 'em," I said, *instead of messing up the titles.*

"Send them to the bakery. Suzy, thanks. You made my day!"

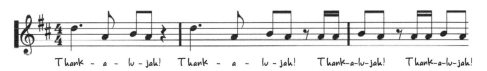

The MRI department was backed up; it'd be at least an hour before they got to me. Waiting takes so much longer when you have nothing (reading, writing, phone calls, etc.) to do. I went up to the coffee shop to investigate the dessert options; then I decided I'd do a complete inventory, which made a trip to the cafeteria on the next floor necessary. I stepped on the elevator with my map; a doctor nodded, and I smiled. *Ha.* I had passed for a healthy person.

I ended up with a coffee and cookie from the coffee shop and returned with my purchases to radiology. I had to avoid looking at the barium swallowers or the coffee thickened in the back of my throat.

"Suzy Becker?" The woman who called my name was holding two johnnies and a pair of slippers. They don't trust anybody with their own outfits. I changed in the bathroom, then waited with another woman in a row of chairs opposite the lockers. "This your first time?" she asked, and I answered no. "Weirdest thing," she said, "all of a sudden, I can't use my right arm. It looks normal—nothing happened to it or anything—but I can't lift a thing. My doctor says it'll go away, but I've got a baby—I can't hold my baby. My husband has to hold the baby. I told the doctor I'm not messing around."

I tried to think of something to say, even if I didn't say it, for practice, so I would have things to say when my speech came back. They were ready for her. "Good-bye!" I meant "good luck," but just as well, since I didn't like it when people in the hospital said it to me.

I had to wait again until the films were ready so I could take them with me to the Brain Tumor Clinic. They called Dr. Finn, and I called Karen (who was meeting me) to let her know I wouldn't get there until 5:15. The directions to the clinic were long and confusing.

what she says:

when you get off the elevator, you want to take the hall that leads to the Chiswick Building, past the...

what I hear:

Take the elevator.

Within a few minutes, I was lost, and beginning to panic.

"Excuse me, where—?" The man didn't even slow down. "Dr. Finn?" A woman stopped at the words "Brain Tumor Clinic," but she had no idea. At that moment, I saw Karen coming to get me.

She gave me a quick hug; then we set off in opposite directions. "I thought you were coming to get *me*," she said. She flagged down a few more people; no one knew where the clinic was. Karen called Dr. Finn's office; a machine picked up since it was after hours.

"Let's go home." I was beyond ready to give up. The next passersby shepherded us onto two more elevators, and we arrived at the clinic at 5:35. The refreshments were gone. We sat down near the front desk where the last two patients were waiting. A fifteen-year-old girl sat facing us in a wheelchair. She could have been one of my old students. Her surgery had partially paralyzed her right side. *That could have been me.* The wheelchair, she explained, was just temporary; they didn't know about the arm. She held it up with her left arm to show us.

Karen asked if she was awake for her surgery. "Oh, no. Were you?" she asked, looking at me. "Oh, my god! What was it like?"—as if being awake were heroic.

A nurse came to get us, and we waited in the back for another half hour. Karen peeked out into the hall. "I wonder if they forgot about us."

"We didn't forget about you!" a nurse yelled out on cue, although she couldn't possibly have heard. "Dr. Finn will be in in just a few minutes."

At 7:15, I got a piece of paper out of the trash and set it down in the middle of the hall.

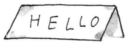

A nurse walked by it. I got a second piece of paper.

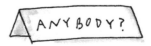

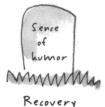

Recovery
Milestone

And a third. The nurse stopped and laughed. She rounded up another nurse and Dr. Finn. He dropped the papers on my lap. "Your sense of humor back?" He smiled.

"Coming."

My MRI showed that a mass of protein and fluid—old blood—was pressing on my brain, causing my difficulties. *So there* was *something!* My brain would reabsorb it over time. "We should give it a couple of months and have another look at an MRI around the first of October. You feeling more like yourself?" Dr. Finn tilted his head, catching my eye.

"Sixly—sixty-five percent."

"Any other troubles? Any more seizures?"

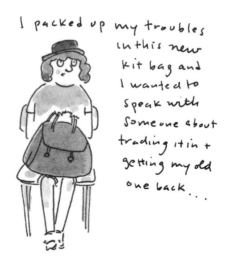

"Headaches. Shaky. Some numb—my right hand. Foot. Jaw hurts." I checked my list. "Um, why do my legs swell?"

"Probably the medication. Do they still?"

"Some. Not as much."

"Been biking?"

"Not. No." *Folks, meet Suzy Becker, the human conversation extinguisher!* "When can I stop Neuron-tin?"

"That's a question for the neurologist. Before I get him, do *you* have any questions?" he asked Karen.

"She's getting back on her bike this weekend. You said this was okay?"

"No wheelies."

"If I'm not better in a year"—I'd practiced while they were talking—"you have to give me a lobotomy—free." Just another option. I could be content sorting silverware on Sunday mornings, if I could forget I used to do the crossword puzzle.

"That right?" He shook his head, backing down the hall.

The neurologist wouldn't let me stop taking the medication. He agreed to see whether he could reduce the dosage, but I was already taking the minimum.

> Egas Moniz shared the 1949 Nobel Prize in medicine for pioneering the lobotomy. The psychological problems produced by the surgery were listed in a monograph he published in 1936; however, he insisted they were transient, lasting no more than several weeks. With absolutely no evidence, he claimed that the surgery did not impair memory or intelligence. The lobotomy is largely discredited and rarely performed today.

It was 8 P.M. when we left the clinic. Karen was quiet when we got back to her place. It had been a long day. A long week. "Are you okay?" I rubbed her head.

Recovery Clock

2 months

"No. Are you?"

I shrugged.

"Two more months. First it was two days. Two weeks. Now it's two months. Aren't you worried—?"

"But this time there's a reason. And it will go away."

"Do you remember my friend Linda LeRoy?" The name was familiar. "She called today about something else, but when she asked how I was, I was telling her about everything, and it turns out she knows this woman, a—see if I get this right—psychoneurophysiologist who runs a center. She started it to help people with cerebral palsy, but now she works with people with all kinds of brain injuries. The idea is, she teaches the brain to repair itself . . . using electrodes. Linda gave me her number, and I left her a message. She's going to call us tomorrow in Bolton. Suz, would you at least talk to her?"

Karen was really worried. *Wasn't that what I wanted from her all along?* It scared me.

The psychoneurophysioelectrodologist returned the call the next day while we were out. I rewound the machine; Karen was standing in the doorway. "I'll call Monday."

"She said she'd be there until two."

"You call her."

Karen took the cordless phone to her chair at the kitchen counter and got out a pad and pen. I sat next to her, in case I was needed at any point during the conversation. After she'd explained my surgery and the outcome, Karen said very little and took notes: 1. Good nutrition. 2. *Arnica montana* reduces swelling. 3. Vitamin E—healing.

I got up and started cleaning the kitchen. Then I gave up on listening and went outside to garden. Forty-five minutes later, Karen burst into the garden. "I'm going to town, I'll be right back!"

"Tell me what she said?"

"Tell you when I get back!" She was trying to hold her mouth straight while the rest of her was smiling. I couldn't remember the last time I'd seen her look happy. Paris? *A hundred years ago.* "I love you." She kissed me and went to her car.

I had gone back to cleaning by the time she got home; she grabbed her pad and led me out to the backyard. "Suz, this is really exciting—just listen, okay? The center is right around the corner from the hospital—she's sure she can make you better. First of all, a lot of what Dr. Finn said is wrong. The brain is a muscle: use it or lose it. The thing about the brain is, is that since there are no pain receptors, you can get to work right away. And the brain wants to work; if it's not working, it's atrophying.

"On the other hand, you should lie low with the physical activity. The stationary bike is okay, but nothing 'jarring or strenuous'—those are her words—because what you could do is stress the arteries. And you don't want any more blood collecting up there. Here, I got you these." A bottle of vitamin E and a plastic vial of *Arnica montana*—they looked like little white love beads. "For the swelling."

"I stopped taking for . . . a week ago."

"I know. She said they don't treat the swelling aggressively enough, which makes total sense, don't you think, since that's what's causing the problem?" I kissed her.

She broke a capsule of vitamin E and rubbed it lightly on my scar. "She does an evaluation, usually takes two to three hours, and then the therapy is set up so you can come in and do it on your own.

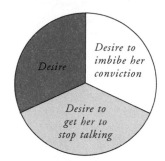

KISSING MOTIVATION

Desire

Desire to imbibe her conviction

Desire to get her to stop talking

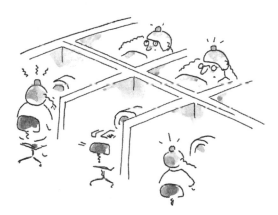

"The evaluation costs two hundred fifty dollars, and after that it's sixty dollars per half hour."

"Does insurance . . . ?"

"None of it's covered. But, if it's the money, Suz, I'll pay." *Am I really that bad?*

"It's not the money. It sounds good. Just scary, a little scary. Electrodes, electricity, *zzzzt,* in your, my brain."

"She has a bunch of studies she's sending you."

"I'll ask Dr. Finn. Maybe if speech therapy doesn't work."

"Why can't you do both?" Karen chucked my chin. "Let's wait and see when we get the stuff."

Ogunquit

8/3

Wow, my writing doesn't get much better-now it's okay. Cripes. It's like I curse it every time I observe it.

Karen and I had our first anniversary. We made love. Coming I felt could tell I'm not all back. I'm beginning to feel interested in sex again. We reminisced about the first year. A lot to love. I still feel like I could love her forever.

I biked 18 miles Sun. Aug 1 - my first day back. I think I did around the same today and I plan to do 20 tomorrow. I figure 25 by this weekend; So by next weekend + 75 for the training ride. I feel a little weak at times.

*O*n my bike, I felt strong. I had no need for words, except "on your right, I mean left, sorry!" *make that* "coming through!" *or* "behind you, thanks!" It was the closest I felt to normal.

I called the speech therapist's office from Maine and got the first available appointment, still a week away. "Is there anything I can do before then?" I asked the scheduler. *Anything to prevent further atrophying?*

"You're in Maine, right? Relax and have a good time!" She gave herself a good laugh.

Karen and I fell into a rhythm of "working" (one to two hours biking, one to two hours work on Ride FAR, for me), breaking for lunch on the porch, then planning our afternoons. If Karen had to do more work on her book, I could decide whether to work, proof her work (a painfully slow, mostly futile attempt to pay down my debt), visit a friend, or rest in the hammock. In the early evening, we walked the dogs. At night, we made trips to the drive-in, had a fried-fish dinner in the canoe, a dinner out in town, and we took our raincheck (from the Fourth of July) on Gabriel's boat.

The day before we left, the man who built Karen's house stopped by. Out of the blue, he said, "I had an MRI. Showed some kind of a mass in my head—they wanted to do surgery. I wouldn't let 'em. I'm sure it's a scar, somethin' from that motorcycle accident I was in." *A scar . . . wouldn't let them?!* "Hey, Karen, have you seen Audrey? She had a stroke."

"Yeah. She's not doing so well. Shame, she was such an intelligent, vibrant woman."

TERRY GROSS: Did you ever worry that people were saying things like that about you?

ME: I guess, when Karen said it. But, that's actually a nice thing to say. When something happens to your brain, people say things—it's this weird open season on your intellect. In case you thought you used to be a genius or something. A couple of people have actually told me they like me better since the brain surgery.

You were never any good at math.

And it's not like you were known for your spelling.

TG: C'mon.

ME: Seriously.

CONUNDRUM COLLASUM

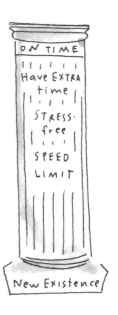

Pillars of My Existence

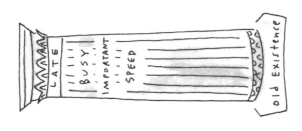

On August 9, one month, one week, and one week-end after my surgery, I had my first appointment with the speech therapist.

I made it all the way to registration before I hit my first snag.

"Your appointment is with?"

"Tim." Once I said it, no last name, it sounded stupid. "In sh-speech."

She peered up at me over the tops of her glasses before leafing through her directory. "Weiland?"

What was the likelihood of more than one Tim in speech? I nodded. She handed me a plastic hospital ID card, and I bristled. *Wallet clutter. This is only temporary.* A vestigial healthy-person reaction.

On the hour, precisely, Tim came down the hall to greet me. He was tall and thin, wearing spectacles and Rockports—the uniform of the People's Republic of Cambridge (as my electrician calls it). His office was a small cube with a window.

TIM'S TINY OFFICE

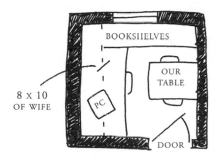

The picture of his wife on his desk was a black-and-white head shot, circa 1980s or '90s, it was hard to tell. She was smiling a wholesome smile, dressed in a turtleneck and sweater, her long light-colored hair pulled back in barrettes. The desk itself was neat. All the papers were in folders, all the folders were filed, all the books were shelved.

Tim opened a new manila folder and creased the spine so it lay flat on his lap. "I know a bit about why you're here, Suzy, but why don't you tell me?" His speech was methodical, not quite slow.

"I hope you can help me"—I felt like Dorothy talking to the Wizard— "with my ssspeech, reading, and writing. Do my work again."

He nodded; he wasn't saying he could. "Tell me about your work." He took notes while I talked—I recognized the informal assessment. I stopped talking, and he looked up.

"Have you worked with other artists before?" I asked him.

"Not an 'artist' per se. I've worked with all kinds of people. We use your work in here: you bring in the stuff you're working on, and we can talk about it. Or, if it's possible, I'll have you do your work here. It doesn't make sense for me to make work. . . ."

It didn't; everybody hates make-work, but there went all my hopes of a magic cure. "Before we can get started, I'm going to have to do some testing."

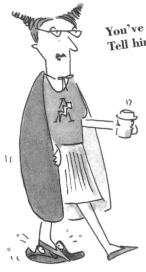

You've already done testing. Tell him you're here to work!

"Unh. Can't you use Dr. Knight's?"

"Unfortunately not. I am required to do my own assessment, partly for insurance purposes. So, the best thing then, I think, is to get it over with as quickly as possible. If we get started now, we can probably finish up next session. When are you scheduled to come back in?" I shook my head. "When would you *like* to come back in?"

"Soon as possible." I picked Friday at 3 P.M. over Friday at 8 A.M., but he hesitated. "Eight, then. I can do eight." He was still hesitating, using up our testing time. "You can to back"—*restart*—"get back to me?"

He put his calendar away and handed me a "Mild Traumatic Brain Injury (TBI) Survey," six pages long.

TESTING?!

How 'bout we do this for homework?

I began. He wrote in my folder. When I was done, we had to go over all the questions on pages one and two orally.

He scanned pages three through six. "Headaches? Have you had those before?" No. "Anxiety?" Well, yes.

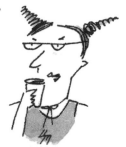

But this is not a figment of our anxiety!

"Irritability?" Mm. "Were you a social person before?" I don't know. *I'm starting to sound like a loser.* "You find it more difficult to be around people? Have you noticed which situations are particularly difficult? For example, some people stop eating out at restaurants; what used to be a pleasant experience is now noisy and distracting for them."

"They do?"

"You don't."

I do! I do! "I thought it was just me. And I can't read the menu, or I can, but then I can't remember what I read. And I hate picking." *I mean ordering.*

"Sure, that's another part of it."

"What else do other people—?" I wouldn't have minded if he spent the rest of the time telling me stories. I had found my people.

"All the things on the survey here, to a greater or lesser extent: paying attention, concentrating for long periods of time—that's probably the biggest complaint." *So, that's what I have, what I've had this whole time, and you've seen it before and you can help me get better and—* "Guilt?"

I cringed. "My mother. Karen. She's given up work, money. I'm not a good partner. Or daughter, sister, friend. Everybody has to do everything for me. I can't do anything for them."

It took him a while to get all that down. "You find it harder or easier to socialize in big groups?"

"Easier." The opposite of what I would have said before. "Less noticing," I meant. "Less people noticing. Less notice if I don't say anything."

"Have you tried to read anything besides the newspaper? A novel or anything?"

"A Widow for One Year."

"How is it?"

"Slow."

"Friends of mine haven't really liked it."

It didn't matter. I couldn't quit my first book.

We were out of time. "I'm not noticing any major difficulties," he summarized. "Mild attention span, stamina. Some of the things you describe with your language are paraphasic errors. The testing should show us some areas to focus on."

Recovery Clock

18 months

"How long will it take?" *To cure me.* September 15 was the first day of the Bunting Fellowship.

"You wrote here you have something, a protein mass that won't clear up until October, right? In my experience, I've seen improvements up to eighteen months." *Eighteen months!!!* "You might want to think of that as a 'recovery window.' I'd be seeing you on a much more occasional basis by then, although we could keep working after that, on certain strategies, improving your memory, for example."

He walked me back down the hall. *Eighteen months?* I'd wanted the real answer all along. "They said one day, then one week, then onth, onth, one month, two months—"

"They do the surgery. I don't think they're trying to mislead you—I'm the one who sees people afterwards. Somebody ought to tell them that it doesn't help to set up—I won't say false—unrealistic expectations. So"—he shook my hand—"very nice meeting you, and I'll call you about Friday."

I stopped by Karen's studio on my way back to Bolton. She was all alone, working at her desk with the lights out and all the fans going. We kissed hello. "How'd it go, your First Day?"

You don't want the truth. "He said eighth, one eight months." She turned away, stared at her desk blotter. I stood there, boardlike.

"What'd you do today?"

"Testing." My board turned into a wet paper towel. She swiveled around and held me on her lap. "He has to start all over again."

"Suz, won't you try the other place I told you about? At least call Dr. Finn and see?" She handed me the phone.

Dr. Finn hadn't heard of it. "Should I try?"

"Should she try?" the nurse repeated. "He says no."

"Give your brain a chance to heal itself." It was Dr. Finn. "Everything else okay?"

"Okay. Thanks." I hung up.

I called Bruce when I got home. He searched "electrode therapy" on the Internet. Not much had been written since the late 1980s. "They said it's like running two hundred twenty vees on a hundred-ten-vee wire," he said, and we laughed—like we're electricians.

A regenerating wire, I thought when I got off the phone. *Had I become less of a risk-taker? I hadn't been afraid of the surgery. Maybe I didn't have a choice.*

Maybe it was like money: my brain didn't like to take risks with money. It'd be different if it were my knee.

But if I really wanted to get better, shouldn't I do it . . . ?

HOW TO GET BETTER

	REST	BIKE	SPEECH THERAPY	ELECTRODES
DR. FINN	●	●		
ME		●	●	
KAREN				●

"I'm going to give my brain six months; after six months, I'll try electrodes," I told Karen.

"It's *your* brain."

She took out pictures her friend had taken on the boat in Maine. My legs didn't look fat in my black swimsuit, but my face—I looked so tentative. Or was that just the way I remembered it? I held the picture up to the refrigerator, next to pictures from before. I used to look more . . . vibrant? My eyes were brighter; my smile, broader. I flipped through the rest of the pile, and the shot on the bottom startled me.

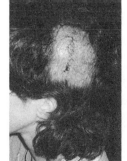

"Scary, huh?" Karen caught me studying that last photograph. Now that I was able to sleep on my scar, and the hair had grown back, the head was a shocker, a mini–medical freak show—more bloodcurdling because it was mine.

That night, I had my first nightmare. They have to go back in. I am on my back, being wheeled into the operating room. The walls are covered in surgical green tile, an old image my subconscious hadn't bothered updating. Dr. Finn is leaning over me; Angela, the nurse, is at my feet. Double doors shut behind us and I want to get off the table, but my arms and legs are somehow fastened, so all I can do is keep turning my head. Shaking my head back and forth so they can't get near it.

The dream woke me up. The sky was light. I checked the clock. *Six. Twenty.* Karen opened her eyes, and I told her the dream. "I don't think I could go through it again."

Our faces are very close together. "You won't have to," she said. And we dozed for another hour.

BROKEN RECORD

I would have said that my progress was indiscernible at the one- to two-month stage, but the weekly check-ins with my therapist marked changes in my thinking, if that could be considered progress.

She began the session. "Did you spend time with Harriet?" *I must have said I was going to.*

"No," I answered. "I feel bad." I'd been one of her most regular visitors at the nursing home. *What if something had happened to her? What if she'd died?* "I feel like I have to put my recovery first." I looked up: *Isn't this one of those statements you're supposed to give me permission to make?*

"How about some of the other questions, who are you without—?"

"Yeah. No. I don't know. I'm spending less time thinking. Makes me sad." The gift of the experience was being wasted on me. I was just trying to get my old unspiritual self back. "I have to do, start cartoons next week." *How are you feeling about that?*

"How are you feeling about that?"

"I'll see. When I sit down."

"You haven't tried?"

"I didn't want to try too early. And fail." She was quiet. "I only need to do two in four weeks."

"For *Grist*?"

I nodded. I had a weekly environmental cartoon on-line and my last batch of ten was running out.

"Did you start speech therapy?"

I grimaced. "Yes."

"Not what you'd hoped?"

"More testing."

She rolled her eyes and took a sip of water. "Did you like the—was it a guy? I don't think you said last time."

"I did, I think, it's hard to tell." All of a sudden there were five things to tell her about at once: *the eighteen-month recovery window; how he didn't have any magic exercises; his uncluttered office and speech; oh, the electrode center, and*—I lost all four trying to remember the fifth and was silent.

"How's Ride FAR coming?"

"I've been riding. I'm up to twenty-fith—shit, sorry—five." *Slow down, Suzy.* "Twenty-five miles. Thirty—seven tomorrow. Fifty this week-end. Seventy-five-mile training ride next weekend."

She reached for her book. "Two weeks?" That'd be my last appoint-ment; another two weeks, I'd be on Ride FAR, and then the fellowship started, September 15.

I missed my next appointment at the rehab hospital. I got there twenty minutes ahead of time, and the parking lot attendant waved me off. "All full."

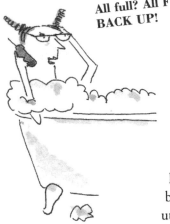

All full? All FULL! Wait a second, BACK UP!

I was back in the middle of Friday (sum-mer) afternoon traffic. The one-way I was on emptied into a rotary, which I circled twice in the middle of a swarm of cars before picking an exit that shot me out over the Charles River, leav-ing downtown far behind. It was 3 P.M., and I pic-tured Tim walking down the hallway. Another ten minutes went by before I found a place I could have turned around (which would have put me back at the hospital at 3:25, leaving twenty-five min-utes for testing, tops). I parked the car a block from Karen's and skulked into a coffee shop. I wasn't ready to deal with her disappointment just yet.

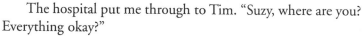

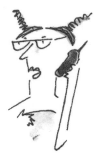

The hospital put me through to Tim. "Suzy, where are you? Everything okay?"

I started to cry. *Lame. Labile.*

"I couldn't park. They said 'full.'"

I could hear him suck his teeth. "I'm sorry. They can't do that to out-patients. Did you tell them—? It doesn't matter. Listen, I want to go talk to someone about this right now. Can I call you back?"

"I'm on the road. To Karen's. Six one seven. Six one seven—" *Dammit. I'm regressing.*

"Call me when you get there. You were my last appointment; I'll stick around and do some paperwork."

I skipped the coffee and went to Karen's. She wasn't home yet, a small relief. I called Tim and took his first opening, plus two more appointments for the following week.

The minute Karen walked through the door, I confessed. Tim made it seem like it was the parking lot attendant's fault.

"Could he do anything about the parking?" she asked.

"If it happens again, I'm supposed to park in the drop-off area and leave the keys with the guard." *I know, another week, no speech therapy.* She didn't have to say anything.

On Monday morning, at 10:40 (two hours and ten minutes later than planned), I began reading the file of environmental news bits I'd stored up. *Step One of the cartooning process.*

I read each paragraph-long story several times for comprehension, then noted any ideas with cartoon potential. In the past, I would have ignored a story I had to read more than once, or indulged a misconception—often the makings for a good cartoon. But that required confidence—almost an arrogance—and lightheartedness. I had neither.

When I got tired of writing, I reviewed my notes. *Useless crap. As if I would recognize cartoon potential—as if I could draw it if I did.* My stomach knotted. *That's what it all comes down to, isn't it?—the drawing.* The knots tightened in affirmation. *The sooner I find out whether I can draw, the sooner I can let the editor know, the sooner he can replace me.*

I had a list of ideas I carried forward from batch to batch in the front of my *Grist* folder. "Recycling confessional: I didn't wash out cat food tins, didn't remove the rings from the bottles, mixed some shiny paper in with my newsprint." The words generally call up a picture in my head, which I realized I must have made up somewhere, but never consciously.

This time I'd have to construct a picture. My head had been ransacked. The kinds of things I'd normally find up there—cartoon ideas, story ideas, random ideas—were gone.

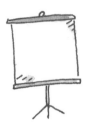 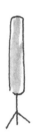 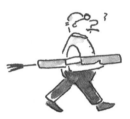

Let's take a brief time out for a pity party: Why can't I have a job where I can fake it and no one would notice? I want to be invisible.

I opened my drawing pad and slipped the cartoon panel outline, a four-by-five-inch rectangle, under the top sheet. I sharpened my blue 2B pencil, collected my erasers (one big and one small), and concentrated on the words. *Recycling confessional. Where you recycle. At the dump. A booth at the dump. A line of people waiting.*

I started with the people; I didn't have to draw them from scratch— *I can recycle them. Ha!* I took out another cartoon and traced the heads. Training wheels, getting the feel back in my drawing hand. I traced the bodies and put the old cartoon away; I gave them accessories—bags and a cart—freehand. Then I made a rectangle booth; all that was left was some background. A desertlike dump with some ash piles and some recognizable refuse. *Not bad.* I held it up next to a cartoon from the last batch. *The heads are a little big, but still, not bad.*

It was 12:30, and I called it a day. An auspicious day. My first day back.

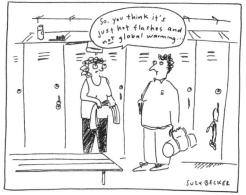

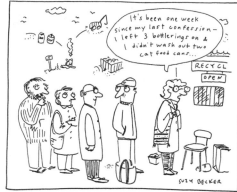

Old batch · New batch

Tim called two days later. He'd had a last-minute cancellation, and he knew I was anxious to finish the testing. I brought the beginnings of my cartoons to show him. He set the testing aside and picked up the papers with the look of an expectant parent.

"Are you having problems with your handwriting?"

"They're *roughs,*" I explained; I don't know what I'd been hoping for in the way of feedback.

He took a longer look. "They're *funny,*" he said, the way people do when they don't generally find cartoons funny. "How do you come up with these?"

The person I'd been waiting all this time to see, who was going to bring me back—the person who was going to help me do my job doesn't even know how to begin to do my job. I *do* know what I was hoping for: "Good start," or, "So then you tighten these up and show them to your editor?"

"Mind if I keep these?" *You really don't get it.* Now he liked them *too* much.

We spent the rest of the session on testing, and he gave me homework: "When I think about going to speech therapy . . ." (Write for ten minutes.)

On August 21, a rainy Saturday, two and a half weeks before the start of Ride FAR, the group gathered at my house for the seventy-five-mile training ride. It was the first time I'd seen or spoken with Meredith in five weeks. Neither of us acknowledged the fact.

She and Jonathan rode just ahead of Randi (a woman I'd been training with) and me. During the first long straightaway, Jonathan pulled away, and we all saw him fork right where the route went left, but none of us could catch him. We waited twenty-five minutes at the fork in the rain, and I started to worry whether we—*specifically I*—could catch up with the rest of the group. (I wasn't used to factoring myself into the group safety equation.) I suggested we go ahead, and Randi agreed, but Meredith wanted to wait.

Five minutes later, we pushed off. *Maybe this'll give Meredith and me time to talk about things.* We rode in silence. Meredith was still mad Jonathan had gone ahead—even after we spotted his jersey. But the second we caught up to him, they made up and rode off together. *It's not just my brain; it's different now. She has him . . . and I have Karen.* We used to be the ones there for each other, but that time was over.

In the afternoon, the route circled back and dumped us out on the same stretch of road. A headwind slanted the cold, light rain toward us. I wished I could go back to worrying about everybody else; worrying about myself only intensified the pounding in my thighs. I concentrated on pulling the pedals up to give my quads a rest. At the seventy-two-mile mark, adrenaline kicked in, and the last three miles flew by.

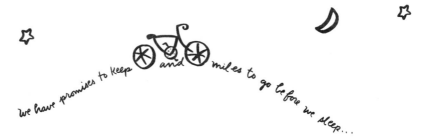

we have promises to keep and miles to go before we sleep...

People were showered when I pulled in the driveway; they already had my grill going. None of them appeared any the worse for my not having worried about them. I leaned my bike against the barn wall, and the exhaustion flooded in. I passed by the crowd in the kitchen and went upstairs to find warm dry clothes. I took an extra minute to sit on my bed. *I haven't had this many people in the house since . . . February.* I just wanted to lie down and wait for Karen.

I scanned the kitchen, looking for a place to sit. On my fourth pass, I realized Karen was back from Maine, engrossed in a conversation at the counter; I waited by her chair. "Excuse me for a second." She held up a finger to put the conversation on hold while she said hello and, "You made it!" She smiled. And I smiled back, remembering when it used to hurt to smile.

Robin, Karen, and I stood by the sink after the house emptied out. "This place is a mess!" Karen grabbed the paper cups and plates off the counter. "I can't believe you let people do this to your house!"

"I wanted them to go." I took the trash out of her hands. "I'll do it."

"They could at least—"

"They offered."

She backed down. "It's not my house."

I went upstairs to shower. There was water all over the bathroom floor. *She was right.*

My dad called while I was showering. "I told him you made it," Robin said, laughing so hard her nostrils were flaring. "Know what he said?" Karen started laughing. *"Sonuvabitch!"*

"No way!"

The three of us cracked up.

K aren and I were lying in bed, finally. I moved over to her side. "What's wrong?"

"Not much of a homecoming," she said. "I came home early to be at your barbecue, and it was like, you could have cared. Suz, we've made love three times since July second—no, since before that because you didn't want to make love in—"

"Sorry. I'm sorry." I rolled back to my side. I fell asleep when I meant to be thinking of what to say next.

T im handed me the homework assignment I had just turned in. "Why don't you read it to me?"

If I had known you were going to ask me, "I never would have written this." I handed it back.

"I'm not sure I understand," he said.

"Too hard to read, for *me* to read—" *Not the reading, too personal.* And it was written in the voice in my head, which had started to come back, but only in my head, not the droning that came out of my mouth.

"You want me to read it?" He started to read without waiting for an answer: "'I was afraid you'd hear me speak and think I didn't need any help and maybe I don't. Maybe my biggest fear is no one can. But you seemed to understand my experiences and you struck me as smart and kind.'" I stared at the picture of his wife; she smiled back. "'I think I still read work-ing or reading comprehension—'" He stopped and started over. "'I think I still read working, read work-ing—'" Like a broken record—

"Need work on! I stopped correcting!"

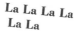

La La La La
La La

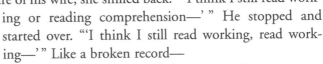

Homework (cont'd.):

I'd like to address my stuttering and reversing sylla-bles. It happens more when I'm tired and under pres-sure. I would like to be able to not have to concentrate so much on the feat of talking so I fun have more fun can have more fun talking again. I'd like to see if my writing (word order, random word endings) could be addressed. I don't know if it's a matter of concentra-tion. Too much concentration can get in the way of what I do. Unlike a lot of work, the less I think about it, the more unpredicatble, broader, looser, better the work is. Back to self-correcting, I think I also need help some strategies for quick decisionmaking, unless the strategy is working out ways so you don't have to make them. I want to feel sharp again. I have trouble staying with conversations and my contributions are off the mark. I was never a know-it-all. I'd like to re-cover the confidence to say I don't know without feel-ing stupid. I say it, but before the surgery I used to say it and still feel smart.

"Well, Suzy," *Yes, Mr. Rogers?* "The good news is we can work on all these things you wrote in here." I rotated my chair ninety degrees and put my legs under the table, indicating my readiness to work. "I have your test results; I thought we'd begin by going over these today."

When do we work?!

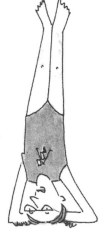

He had a handout that explained the relationships between the raw scores, the percentiles, and the normal curve equivalent. *Normal on a scale of "Does two pounds of flour— ?"* I didn't need a college-educated normal curve; I just needed some perspective. We used up the rest of the time going over his performance summary. The next time, he promised, we'd work.

I had an appointment with my therapist in between the two appointments with Tim. My last.

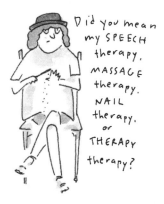

Did you mean my SPEECH therapy, MASSAGE therapy, NAIL therapy, or THERAPY therapy?

I knew I needed to do more work *(doesn't everybody?)*, but speech therapy was beginning in earnest, and then the fellowship. I said very little; the farewell scene loomed.

When the bird finally called on the hour and my therapist flipped her appointment book open to September, I said, "I was thinking, I'll just call when Ride FAR's over." But then I never did.

That was some farewell.

The next time, when Tim escorted me back to his office, he stopped to introduce me to the director. The meeting—her handshake alone (cold and limp)—ruled out the possibility of going over his head.

"I think I know about the visual recall," I said somewhat abruptly after I sat down. I had stopped using people's names or introductory phrases—fewer words. "I'm not looking long enough. It used to be long enough, but it's not now." I'd figured it out when the person I thought was my blond friend Catie biking toward me turned out to be a much older dark-haired man. Tim's performance summary had given my self-observation and analysis new focus. "I *think* I have it, so I stop looking, then I find out I don't have it at all. I do it all the time, I didn't notice it before—with signs, faces, if I reach for something on a shelf—"

"So . . ."

"So, I have to look longer. Until it comes back."

"In a sense, what you're saying is, you have to slow down. People used to doing things very quickly have to learn to s-l-o-w-w-w down." *You aren't one of us, are you?* "I have to write up a formal evaluation of my assessment and interview later this afternoon, but I wanted to let you know, I am diagnosing your difficulties as 'mild.' I hope that's okay." He was apologizing for labeling me 'mildly brain-injured,' not for downplaying the severity of my difficulties. Either way, I didn't care, as long as we could get started. "They've already authorized the first six visits; I'm asking for six more—we can go over all of this next time. I'll have a copy of my report for you." *I don't need a copy of the report, can't we please—?* "After the twelve, we'll have to do more testing—"

"Tim, can we start?"

He transferred my folder from his lap to the table and pulled up his chair. "I thought we'd begin by looking at some of the difficulties you are experiencing, let's say, with your work—see if there are any patterns, maybe group things together, prioritize, and if we have time, go over some strategies."

"I wrote about my difficulties Month, Monday." *I am tired of talking about my difficulties. And testing. And results. I am tired of talking in a CALM VOICE when all this time is TICKING away.* "I *really* want to start. To *do* something.

Today. To have *real* homework. Didn't the tests tell you"—*I don't mean to*—"what to do next?"

"The trouble is, there are no real patterns to your language problems—none that I've been able to detect. If you had problems saying certain words, if certain sounds were difficult, it'd be real easy to pull out pronunciation exercises. A lot of people, for example, have trouble with pronouns."

"I do."

"That's actually not a good example; pronouns are a matter of practice and self-correction. You already do that. Many people aren't aware of the problem." He hesitated. "I should tell you, Suzy, some of these things don't go away." *Self-correction is as good as it gets?* "You have to learn to deal with them. Whereas you might've been comfortable speaking off the cuff before, you'll need to write things out and go over them first. We can do that here; I can help you identify the tough spots and we can practice until you're comfortable." *And then I get back to speaking off the cuff?*

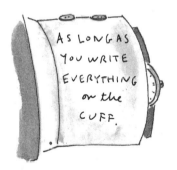

"How about my numbers? And why do I blurt out colors when I mean something else?"

"Interesting." He cocked his head. "There's a lot we don't know. How's the Irving book; do you like it?" *I told you last time.* "Friends of mine haven't liked it." *You told me last time.*

I wasn't going to have any speech breakthroughs by giving my therapist the silent treatment. "I understand what I read. Mostly. Sometimes I miss words or lines. I don't know if it's my attention span or my eyes, you know, looking-not-looking." I was searching for the word *tracking.* "The way my eyes used to move before, like the picture recall thing; they are moving too fast to read."

"Probably both."

"I can't remember my point."

"You're having trouble tracking when you read."

I knew how to fix that: slow down. "If I put the book down, I can't remember what I read."

"Your memory has been impacted. You will need to help it along, create what we call 'memory tags.' When you come to the end of a chapter, I want you to write down—you can keep a five-by-seven card right in the book, use it as a bookmark—make a few notes about the plot. Number one: the plot," he repeated. "Number two: any new characters. The plot, any new characters, and number three: a couple of sentences about what you think will happen next." *A prediction.* I gave myself homework: Record language problems to see if there are any patterns.

"You might think about joining a book group. We have one here at the hospital for our patients.

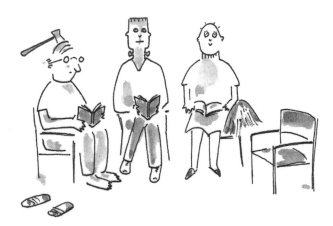

"Or you could find one on your own. Our time today, unfortunately, is up, and I didn't see you on my schedule."

"Next week is pretty busy, and Ride FAR is the week after that. Then the Bunting—"

"So, you've made up your mind to do it." It didn't have the ring of "sonuvabitch."

"Try."

"I'll be very eager to hear how it all goes. Keep me posted."

Did he think this was good-bye? "I'll call when I know my schedule."

I dialed Alyson Caldwell's number. "Alyson, it's Suzy Becker, Cathy Freed's . . ." She knew. "This a bad time? You in a meeting or—?" She shut her door so we could talk. "I started shpeech"—I *had* to laugh—"therapy. And I don't know. Yours sounded much better." *Or maybe you were a better patient. More patient.*

"You have to be really firm. Tell them what's working and not working. It shouldn't be a waste of time." *Nothing's working; there is no working.* "I can give you the name of the person I worked with; I don't know if she's still there." I took the number. "How's everything else?"

"Good. I mean better." *You know.* "It's hard."

"Yeah. You have to take it really slowly. Some stuff must be coming back, right? It doesn't happen overnight. Like I said last time, you've got a head start. Just be patient."

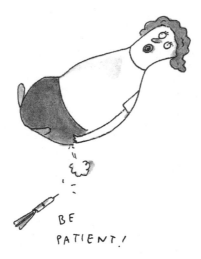

BE
PATIENT!

SONUVABITCH!

The night before Ride FAR I went to bed at 2:00, not bad compared with Ride FARs one through five, only bad considering my alarm was set for 5:30 A.M.

I woke up around 3:30. My skin felt like it was tightening around my skull, the way it used to when I felt a seizure coming on. I turned on the light. *I cannot have a seizure now. Go away! I am AWAKE.*

I wished Karen were there. *I can't stay awake. I have to sleep. I have to bike a hundred miles.* I turned off the light. *I can't sleep.* I put the light back on. I felt delirious; the tightening skin felt like crawling, like things were crawling under my skin. *Maybe it's infected. Maybe I'm bleeding again. Maybe they didn't get it, and this is really it, The End. I have to call Karen.*

I stood up to get the phone. *I can't call Karen; she won't let me on my bike.* I turned the lights back off and lay on my side, pressing my forehead into Karen's pillows. I put another pillow on top of my head and rested in my pillow cocoon until it was time to get up.

After I showered, I walked out into the morning darkness. *One little prayer: God, or whoever, please, no seizure today. Not on the first day of this trip, not in the first six months. I promise I will get more rest. Please?*

The morning darkness never completely lifted. It molted into gray. The riders and crew arrived, unloaded their bags and bikes. Karen was snapping pictures. There was a current in the air, rain on the way. Prerace jitters.

I met with the road crew to go over the day's logis-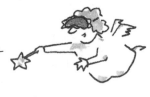
tics. By 7 A.M., the check-in table was folded up and
loaded into the van. Everybody was gathered, and I
began the general safety talk. My voice had retreated back to my throat. I moved on to the par-
ticulars of the day's route, passed out the cue sheets.

Your delivery fits the subject matter...

The worst of the talking was over. *Then, how come I
don't feel any less nervous?* For the first time in ten years, I was nervous about
riding again.

The first day was one hundred miles through the hills of central
Massachusetts, ending up in the northeast corner of Connecticut.
Everybody was in good spirits at the morning rest stop, an apple orchard
twenty-five miles out.

A cold rain began falling during the next twenty-five. I started to worry
about the lack of cover at the lunch stop—until I reminded myself not to
worry. *Hey, you haven't worried about having a seizure since you got on your
bike!* I'd completely forgotten the night before.

The picnic area was tented, and the road crew had set out hot coffee,
tea, and cocoa alongside our donated lunches. There were signs of weari-
ness—people shivering absentmindedly, rejecting advice to put on extra
clothes until a sweatshirt was held out to them.

The twenty-five miles after lunch are always the hardest—not the ter-
rain, but the fatigue. Knowing you still have another twenty-five to go after
that. You can ignore the accumulated soreness, the way your seat refuses to
get comfortable in the last twenty-five. Just when you are ready to let yourself believe they are the hardest twenty-five, the end reels you in.

There were no turns to mark miles ninety-four through one hundred,
and I don't cycle with an odometer, but I'd been keeping an eye on my
watch. *It can't be more than thirty more minutes.* I resisted checking my
watch until twenty-five minutes had gone by, and when I looked back up,
I could see the SLEEP INN sign lit against the still gray sky. *I made it.* The
lead in my legs turned lavalike, swirling. I firmed my grip on the handlebars. "Yes!"

The back road went past the travel plaza to the parking lot, where it
merged with the car and truck traffic exiting the highway. I wove my way

around the eighteen-wheeled Goliaths, the opening car doors, to the finish. I didn't see who took my bike away. I was wobbly without it, and the next thing I knew, Robin's arms were around me. "You made it, you sonuvabitch!"

We were laughing, tears streaming, and then I started to shudder, from the cold and exhaustion, the two months of pent-up uncertainty. Robin handed me a copper disc with *100* stamped in the center to put on my silver chain. My hands were too shaky to open the catch. As she reached around my neck, I heard Meredith say, "Is Suzy in? . . . Oh, yes! " I turned toward her; her face was quivering.

CAN-DO

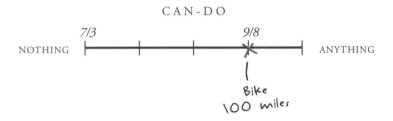

Karen pulled up in the trail van. She ditched unpacking to find me. "Oh, my god, you're here! You made it! You're okay. I am *wiped!* I was *so* worried. I have to go to the bathroom—what are you smiling at?"

"You." I wanted her to go on and on. . . . "I love you."

By the next morning, somebody had replaced my water bottle with a Stone Cold Steve Austin action figure water bottle. *Nice memento.* I filled it. *No nervous stomach.* My old riding confidence was back, paired up with my new "what good did worrying about them ever do?" attitude.

Miles 101 to 200 were uneventful. That night's accommodations were deluxe. The thirty-five of us were eating pizza around the hotel pool. *This might be the best part of Ride FAR.* The little community we become; everybody at their best for five days, a sustainable period of time.

The third morning, it was pouring, hardly any light at all. When we rode out to breakfast, I whittled my usual rain-riding safety speech down to one line, the least obvious:

"Remember to drink. One bottle an hour. Even when you're wet and cold."

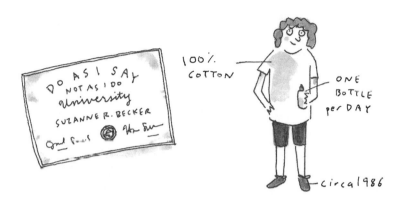

A mile from the first rest stop, I was thinking about how the rain was going to wreck our walk-up concert ticket sales that night. . . . *Good thing we sold a lot in advance . . . Bruce's parents are probably on their way to pick up our cookies—* BAM! I was down. I'd taken slick railroad tracks at an angle and landed on my flank, still holding on to the handlebars, my toes clipped into my pedals. Luckily, other riders were far enough behind so I didn't take them out, too. And I didn't hit my head. No one saw me; I was up in no time. The damage was minimal; my handlebars were slightly bent, but the wheels were fine. And there was a lot of blood from a tiny cut on my ankle. *Just a wake-up call.*

Under normal circumstances, a near miss would have compelled me to expand on my earlier safety speech. I was still feeling shaken and said nothing when we got to the bagel place.

The next stretch was a long one: thirty-seven miles to my mother's lunch stop. The rain was showing no signs of slowing. Fifteen miles out, we were in the center of Andover, and I saw the lead van parked. Road-crew members were flagging traffic so riders could safely cross, but, five minutes after I crossed, I realized I (and everybody ahead of me) was now ahead of the lead van. I stopped.

Laura's group caught up to me. "Everybody okay?" she called out as she rolled by.

Not sure? "No! Stop! Wait. The lead van has to go first."

"Wait in the rain?" Laura asked. *Do I detect an "are you crazy?" in your tone?* "Isn't the route marked? Aren't there other people ahead of us?

Stop questioning my judgment and dismount!

"Want me to ride ahead and catch them?"

"NO! No, I don't want anyone riding alone." *Van, appear! My brain damage is showing—inflexible, unable to consider other options, clinging to my rules . . . Please, van! My mother is waiting with sandwiches at a park in the rain.*

I held up another group of riders. After fifteen minutes, they were all getting to me—the disapproving silence, the glares, the cold. "We're going to go ahead using the tag system. Two at a time. Laura's group can start out. Wait for the next two at the turn. Wait if you have any questions."

Classic mismanagement: setting limits, then changing them. I am putting the group at risk.

Randi and I went last; we were waiting at the first turn when the lead van raced past. Flagging them would only have slowed things down. It was a long twenty miles to lunch, hoping no one was lost or hurt.

Everyone was fine. And the rain took a break. My mother was posing for photos in her rain gear, surrounded by riders. I went to find Bill, the head of the road crew and driver of the lead van. "That can't happen again," I said (no hello) with my helmet still on. "No riders ahead of the lead van." I continued to bark pygmy sentences. "If you stop, they stop."

Bill was soaked. Not fazed. I went on, "Especially in the rain. We can't have people riding extra miles." No response. He didn't bother to explain the cell phones were out of range and the vehicle that should have taken his place was held up, fixing flats. "In the rain," I sputtered, out of steam.

"You okay? Need a sandwich? Dry clothes? Something?" he asked.

"I'm going to go say hello to my mother." I suddenly felt sheepish.

My mother was receiving compliments on her legendary "power muffins." I hugged her just as the trail van pulled in; Karen jumped out to grab a couple of sandwiches, and they pulled back out.

"The trail van should *never* pass the last riders!" I barked at the exhaust. *The system is breaking down; I've lost control.*

After lunch, it rained harder, as if it had been saving itself up during the break. We had to hold up under a strip mall overhang, the third rest stop; at least half the group's brake pads needed replacing. Steamy sheets of rain swept across the parking lot; the drops were visible only when they bounced off a car or helmet. Riders sang shower-style as they pedaled out again.

I was coasting down a hill, two miles from the end, when I saw Kevin holding up his hand, yelling, "Stop!"

"Stopping!" I yelled to warn the riders behind me.

"Walk," Kevin said, once we'd stopped. His lips were white. "The bridge is metal—three of us fell—we're lucky there was no car." *"Walk across metal bridges," from Ride FAR Rain-Riding Safety Talk, the unabridged version.* Robin had stopped in the middle of the bridge—*danger!*—with her emergency lights flashing. *Focus.* Kevin's cheek was bruised. His lips were shaking.

"Kevin, let Randi tell people to stop. You need more clothes." I walked him to the car.

"Tammy's hurt pretty bad; Shari and Mike are okay, I think—they kept going. I'm okay," he said, and looked over at me.

"Your bike?"

"Fine." He was shaking his hand.

"That"—I caught the hand—"doesn't look good." He took it back.

Five people hovered around the back of Robin's car in the middle of the road. (Laura and Tammy were already inside.) Only one person was needed to load the bikes on the back; the rest belonged on the sidewalk. "Rob"—I could see the panic on her face—"you need to get Tammy to the hospital. The church is up on your right, send Laura in for directions. Have Tammy's medical form ready."

The rest of the riders walked across the bridge. When I got to the church, Kevin was wrapped in blankets, icing his hand. An egg had come up on his cheek. I handed him a bowl of chili.

Shari came back from showering; her finger was crooked. "I do *not* want medical attention," she said without slowing down.

I waited until she was seated, and I slipped an ice pack under her palm. "Twenty minutes on, twenty minutes off. I'm going to ask for a doctor from the stage and have your finger checked at intermission."

"I'm riding." *Are you testing me?*

I grabbed a ride to the showers. There were flood advisories on the radio. My driver talked in torrents, undeterred by the rain, my response-lessness, or by the fact that we were lost and the concert was starting in ten minutes. I interrupted: "I think we should go back."

She knew the Y was around there somewhere. I gave her another minute. "It's okay, I have to get back." She was silent. I prefaced my thank-you with a sorry, then ran to change my clothes in the church kitchen. The dinner was gone. There wasn't much of a crowd for the concert, and no word yet from the hospital.

Karen was shooting pictures of the first performer with the AIDS Memorial Quilt hanging behind her. I sat alone in the back; riders and road crew were seated with friends, laughing and clapping. I could have been watching the whole thing on TV.

Robin tapped me from behind. "I'm back."

"How's Tammy?"

"She's going to be fine. The X rays were all fine."

> I am not a passenger,
> I am the ride.
>
> —CHRIS SMITHER,
> "THE RIDE"

Just before intermission, the emcee called all the Ride FAR participants up to the stage. As he announced that we were still waiting for one more rider, Laura and Tammy walked through the door. The audience applauded. During intermission, two doctors gave Kevin and Shari the okay to ride. The house seemed fuller once everyone was in, safe and sound.

Robin, Karen, and I shared a room at the host family's house. I heard the two of them talking from the shower. My arms and legs were plastered with dirt, chain grease, and blood from my fall, a million miles ago. The ankle was bruised, but not too swollen. *I should have at least said something about the tracks. It could have saved us from the rest.*

RESTART The next morning, the fourth day, the sun was out. The air was cool, fall-like. Everything washed clean by the rain. All twenty-five of us were back on our bikes. An easy hundred miles on the coast, up into New Hampshire.

The last day, I caught sight of our motorcycle escorts at the 490-mile mark—their horns going, their Ride FAR banners whipping in the wind. Tears mixed with sweat in the hair at my temples. *You really thought you couldn't do it, didn't you? I didn't let that stop me from doing it. You'd done it five times already. I had brain surgery, let me have this one.*

My speech was shot. I should have saved some words for the closing dinner. "Our final total is one thousand, one hundredth, one thou"—One last try, slowly—"one hundred fourteen thousand dollars." We topped the last ride's total by twenty-five thousand dollars.

There was a long ovation. *I wonder if it was the brain surgery . . . No second craniotomies, not even for this cause . . .* The group presented me with a gift certificate to the bakery for $214.

F

½

E

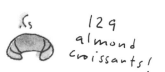

Is   12 9
almond
Croissants!

Le GRAND CIRCLE

Karen and I slept late, then we headed in to Cambridge in separate cars. It was move-in day at the Bunting Institute.

Rediscovery was the best part of my recovery—the way it made things new again. If I was careful, I could sometimes keep the window of newness open, keep the familiarity from rushing back in. Setting up a new office was a chance to see how I worked, exactly what I needed. I had a small box with me, two handfuls of office supplies. I planned to move in in stages.

OFFICE NEEDS

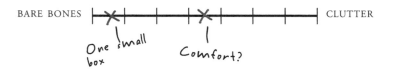

I walked into the main building on Concord Avenue, where I'd dropped off my application almost a year before. The receptionist's desk was empty; a WELCOME '99–'00 FELLOWS! sign sat in her place. Several more signs were posted in the lobby area. Keys were being given out in the library, one fellow at a time.

I waited in a wing chair with my back to the library—*"startled" isn't a good first impression*—and then switched to the opposite chair. Ditto *"idle."* I picked up the Harvard newspaper.

Recent graduate Anne-Marie Oreskovich of Spokane, Wash., is currently studying for a Ph.D. in mathematics at University of California at Los Angeles. Besides being an outstanding mathematician, Oreskovich is a gifted opera singer, a nationally ranked tennis player, a published poet, a musical composer, a marathon runner, and a hospital volunteer. As a result of her grandmother's death from cancer, Oreskovich has resolved to pursue a career in the cutting-edge science of mathematics at the Centre for Mathematical Biology, Oxford University, one of the only two centers in the world specializing in this.

The library door opened. I dropped the newspaper and got up to meet my first fellow. She pivoted at my old chair and walked out the front door without so much as a sideways look in my direction.

The director stood to introduce herself and her assistant. I introduced myself. *Suzy,* all of a sudden, sounded so unacademic. The assistant slid a pocket folder across the conference room table. "Everything you need to know"—*a reference to my book?*—"and your keys." *No.*

"Any questions? Anything you need from us?" the director asked.

I couldn't think of anything, but there *had* to be something; the first fellow had been in there for at least twenty minutes. Someone barged in the door behind me. It was First Fellow.

"Excuse me. There's no phone in my office." *All the literature said "no phones." Even I-of-limited-reading-comprehension understood that.*

"We can have one installed for you by the university," the director offered, and the assistant made a note to set it up. I dumped out the miniature manila envelope in my palm and stared at four identical keys.

First Fellow wasn't finished: "Meanwhile, there are things I have absolutely no use for: a *typing* table, enough filing cabinets for an army, and a hideous armchair . . ."

"If you'll let us know what you don't want, we'll have someone take it down to the basement," the director said with a smile. I decided against introducing myself to First Fellow. She shut the door after herself. And, click, their smiles went off. Not a single eye rolled.

"Well, thank you." I thought I'd aim for the opposite end of the entitlement spectrum. "I wanted to thank you for the"—*not fellowship, what's the word?*—"um, chance. Chance to be here." They stood, and I let myself out. No one else was waiting.

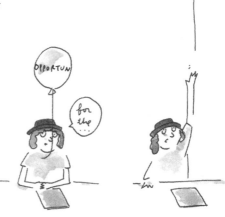

M y office was in the building next door—the one with the typing table (had to be First Fellow's) sitting on the lawn in front. I stood on the stairs of the main building and sorted my keys; *no fumbling in front of First Fellow.* But my timing was such that no key was necessary—the hideous armchair was coming through the door. I held it open and peeked my head around as it went by. "Suzy Becker."

"Myra Goldsheid." End of conversation. I stepped into the building, and there was her name, first door on the left. My office was not one but two doors down.

> **Suzy Becker**
> **Nonfiction**

Creative writing, *not* nonfiction. *Mistake, little mistake.* I'd have to bring it to someone's attention lest people think I was doing research or something serious in there.

Otherwise, I was thrilled with my new office. It had windows on three sides. A couch that matched the hideous armchair (hardly offensive compared with some of the special orders I'd seen leave my dad's furniture factory). More important, it was big enough to lie down on. A desk, also big enough to lie down on. A typing table. Three incandescent lights positioned so that I'd never have to use the fluorescent overhead. And a piano. I put my box on my desk, pulled my shades halfway up, and left. *I had my own office. At Harvard.*

I stopped back at the library on my way to the car. I set my nameplate down on the lacquered conference table and said, "My office is great, just that, um, I'm a fellow in Creative Writing."

"All of our writers are creative," the director cooed. "What's your project again?"

I still couldn't say *illustrated* reliably.

"Memoir. With art. Baby decision."

"Well, that would be nonfiction, right?"

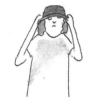

\.

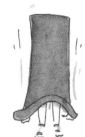

2.

I let myself back out, sure there was eye-rolling this time.

Two mornings later, Karen and I were having coffee and cereal while my sister fellows were mingling over continental breakfast, the first day of our official orientation. "I better go." Karen nodded. It was the fifth time I'd said it. "Okay, this is really it." She waited to see if I was going to sit back down before she stood.

"You look very cute, and I'm proud of you." She stepped back. "No hat?"

I shook my head. Truth was, I'd stopped needing a hat to cover the incision in late August, but I'd kept wearing it to hide my bad hair. To hide, period. It was time to give up the hat. "We have a group photo," I explained as I kissed her good-bye.

I got to the Bunting with enough time to find my name tag and take a seat next to one of the science fellows. "You were smart," she said. "I wish I'd worn jeans."

I was the only one wearing jeans. And if it had escaped anyone's notice, at 10:15, the photographer asked us to arrange ourselves by height, "except *you*, let's hide you in the middle somewhere."

I was late to the next official session, "Introduction to Colloquia." It was pouring, reminiscent of the Ride FAR Friday. *Was it just the week before?* I spotted my science fellow, in jeans, and sat down next to her again. She was taking notes, "Purpose of colloquium—threefold." I opened my notebook.

Concerning the podium, the presenter said, "I encourage you to take your watch off and lay it flat here, rather than looking at it every five minutes. We will have fresh water for you, or you may choose to bring your own. Another piece of advice—" She poured a glass, placed it on the podium, and we all watched it slide down. "Place it underneath." People, *extremely smart people,* were making a note of this. She moved on to audiovisual aids. "I don't want anybody standing up here and using PowerPoint for the first time."

During that awful, painfully serious session, my mind felt the glorious urge to wander again.

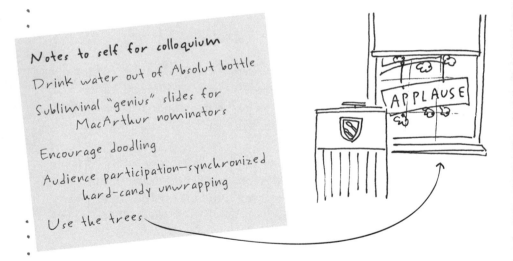

Karen and I were looking at the paper on Sunday night, getting ready to go to bed. "Think we can sleep in the loft tonight?" she asked. "It's cool enough." I was so used to sleeping downstairs, I'd forgotten all about the loft. Karen carried Molly, and I climbed up after the two of them. Mister harrumphed down below and then settled into an oversize armchair.

I broached another subject. "Volleyball starts this week."

"You're not playing. What if you get hit on the head?"

"I won't." It happens maybe once a season. "If Dr. Finn says it's okay?" We both knew what Dr. Finn would say.

"If his nurse says it's okay."

"So, then"—this was the part I'd figured out, the part I was excited to tell her—"I'll come on Thurs—I mean—Tuesdays after volleyball and stay through Friday. Then we can decide where we want to spend the weekend, in—"

"Wait, are you asking me or telling me?"

Asking hadn't crossed my mind. "This—" *Goddammit, I wish I had all my words. This is what we've been looking forward to. This is what we dreamed about when I applied to the Bunting—*

"My place isn't big enough for the two of us with two dogs. It's a crash pad."

Then what am I (and my dog) doing here? I cried and cried. (It had been a relatively long time since I'd cried.)

"You're overreacting. This doesn't change anything."

Does, too. But I couldn't explain it to her.

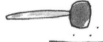

Our future

I went downstairs and slept beside Mister. The next morning, I didn't feel like breakfast. Or a dog walk. Or saying "I love you," which wasn't the same as not loving her, but I wasn't even going to give her that. I just wanted to go. Not to the Bunting. Home.

I called Dr. Finn's nurse from my studio. She counted off the months—three—since the surgery. "I think volleyball's okay. Concussion's the worst we're talking here, right? You're no more at risk than the next person, and if anyone tells you to wear a helmet—tell them to forget it. A helmet is meant to absorb the impact of a crash, not a ball. It would actually make things worse—it's harder than a ball." *I'd play in a dress before I'd play in a helmet.*

The first practice was everybody's first night back, the first night of the indoor volleyball season. I hadn't touched a ball since the day before my MRI. I trusted my brain and muscles enough that the physical part didn't make me nervous anymore. (Whistling, swimming, and biking had all come back.) I *was* afraid of getting hit in the head, which meant I was constantly looking behind me. My neck was stiff, maybe from bracing my head on the bike all month; I could hear it pop each time I followed the arc of the ball.

"Is that someone's *neck?*" the coach asked. "Man, let me give you some stretching exercises after practice."

I couldn't run the offense; I couldn't read the whole court, yell out a player's name, or a play number or some one-word command with any accuracy. I simply reacted to the ball and put up the easiest (not the best) set, but no one seemed to notice.

They call their own plays anyway...

I stayed at Karen's after practice. *Maybe it didn't change anything.* Wednesday was my first full day at the Bunting.

SCHEDULE	
10:30 A.M.	Colloquial dinner beverage shopping with Liz-the-poet
11 A.M.	E-mail info session
12 NOON	Meet with communications director
1 P.M.	Meet with associate director
4 P.M	Liz's colloquium, colloquial dinner

"My goal," the communications director told me, "is to get each one of you at least one interview or one published piece." She paused. "With most fellows, it's obvious from their projects or CVs—I wanted to ask you, what *is* your area of expertise? It helps to know when I'm searching around or if I get calls."

Like Harvard expert? "Could I get back to you?" As if that hadn't answered her question, I added, "Um, I don't know if you know, knew, but, I had brain surgery in July. I am not ready to do interviews." *Who knows, you may get an inquiry for a real dolt.*

But afterwards, I couldn't let the question go; I had to come up with an answer, no longer for her—for myself. *Small business, entrepreneurship, the greeting card industry, charter schools? Expertise, not outdated experience.* I wasn't a writer like the other Bunting writers. Or an artist like the artists. (I'd noticed that whoever prepared our bios in the class booklet had bulked up my education by running my two B.A.s on separate lines. Two more areas—international relations and economics—in which I am also not an expert.) *This is an identity crisis you have had before. And are not ready to have now.* I let it go.

I QUIT!

Renny, the associate director, inquired about my health at our meeting. She was much more of the housemotherly type. I confided in her how intimidating it was to be there. My eyes were tearing up.

"Harvard's an intimidating place. There are fellows who have this problem every year." She lowered her glasses. "I don't know what else I can tell you." She slid the glasses back up her nose. "Now, how can I help you?"

I couldn't think how. I guess I should have expected the question.

"Is there someone you'd like to meet?" She reeled off a list of authors. *It's not that I don't want to meet them, but meetings have never been and now are certainly not my best medium. I would do much better with something nonverbal—a bike ride or ping-pong. What would we meet about, anyway?* "Well, if you think of something."

"I'll try to, thanks."

I did. I picked up a course guide at lunch and went back to her office. The guide was easily two inches thick; I'd never get through it. Perhaps she could point me in a direction. "Do you have any ideas?" *Recommendations* (polysyllabic word avoidance). "Any subject, as long as the professor is good. The lecture, I mean."

"You're going to have to narrow it down."

"Philosophy. Religion. Lit, American."

She recommended a course taught by the poet Helen Vendler.

I made several attempts to take Helen Vendler's course.

Attempt #1   No info on-line.
Attempt #2   Call information for English department telephone number.

Attempt #3	Call English department; told to call back with course number.
Attempt #4	Told to call back with catalog number; different from course number.
Attempt #5	Call back; told that course not being offered this year.
Attempt #6	Call back with another catalog number. This course info is on-line.
Attempt #7	Go to class; room is empty except for visitor from Israel who also read about class on-line.
Attempt #8	It is raining on day of next scheduled class. Give up.

The orientation room was completely filled for Liz-the-poet's (our first) colloquium. The director gave an embarrassingly long introduction, beginning with citations from glowing reviews and an enumeration of Liz's degrees (after which she was referred to as Dr. Arnold), a full three minutes on her publications, prizes, and then her language proficiencies. *Note to self: Tell associate director about French and conversational Spanish. She is going to need filler.*

The crowd—a Cambridge poetry crowd—was very receptive, in their poetry way, to Liz's work.

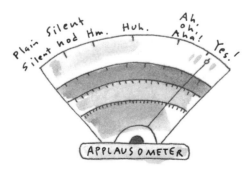

CALIBRATED for POETRY CROWD

I made a quick exit before the Q&A to meet the dinner delivery person and set out the food as I'd promised Liz. A couple of dozen fellows and guests came downstairs for dinner after the Q&A, and we were introduced to the Bunting dinner rituals: a celebratory toast and the passing of the "cost-sharing experience" basket. The phrase "cost-sharing experience" elicited snickers—I paid particular attention to what the group found funny. We weren't often on the same funny wavelength, which didn't bode well for my work, *if I ever begin it.*

The colloquium experience didn't end with dinner; there was a brown bag lunch the next day, attended by a smaller group—some fellows and one or two guests. The lunch serves the second fold of the threefold colloquium purpose, the "reality check." The fellows tell you what they *really* think of your "work-in-progress." Except, or as a result, most people, like Liz, presented from already published works—a fairly bulletproof reality.

The lunch discussion revolved around some of the more obscure allusions in Liz's poetry, which led me to conclude that the actual subject, her lymphoma as an adolescent, was too personal, which also did not bode well for my work, should I start. And I'd need to beef up the obscure references.

I waited for Liz when the lunch was over. She said she wished it had gone better. I couldn't think what to say. "Wanna go for a dog walk?" I tried to think of consolations on the drive to the pond.

"You must be relieved," was all I came up with. She shrugged. The dogs had decided to trespass on the golf course.

Once we were a safe distance from the green, I told her I'd had brain surgery, by way of an explanation or excuse for my failure to come up with anything else. She couldn't believe it was just this summer. I changed the subject back to her. "Do you have to worry about your cancer coming back?"

"Not the lymphoma, but I have to worry about all these other cancers. The side effects from having so much radiation in my teens."

Just then the dogs went airborne, tackling each other. We laughed out loud and continued walking.

When we got back, the fellows were assembling outside for the "Grand Circle," the conclusion of our Bunting Orientation.

No one knew what a Grand Circle was, and none of us (with all our achievements) had dared to ask.

Forty women, including staff, were seated in a large circle. A small basket of stones sat on the grass in the very middle.

The director explained the ritual: this first circle was a way of getting to know each other, something a résumé wouldn't tell us. We were supposed to say our names and tell a story about ourselves, because "as women, we have a great tradition of storytelling. This is how we talk to each other while we cook; we love to gossip." Everybody got a prize for telling a story, a special stone (collected by fellows over the years) from the basket.

The director started things off. I don't remember a single word of her story, just that it managed to portray her intelligence, strength, courage, and compassion with humor and humility. She set the bar *very* high.

A few others who had stories at the ready went next. Then we hit our first silence. Myra broke it. "I think all this community stuff is a crock, and it would be completely hypocritical for me to participate." She didn't get a stone.

A writer went next. "I hate these things, too, and I'm a storyteller. People lay this stuff out there, and you feel like you're supposed to get up and wrap a blanket around them. . . . I pass, too."

The mood shifted from hostile to what-the-hell, go-and-get-it-over-with. Normally I would have gone in this round. There were a couple of times when I thought of a connection, a logic as to why I'd go next, but I still didn't have a story. *Here's something to work on in speech therapy: saying more than the bare minimum.* I hadn't told a story since the surgery. Not to one person, much less a group.

There were just a handful of us left. Pat, whose office was opposite the bathroom, diagonally across from mine, went. "Well, I have to go pick up my son, so I can't put this off much longer. I really don't have a 'story'"— her eyes were watery—"it's more about where I am. A year and a half ago,

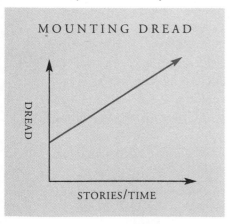

MOUNTING DREAD

DREAD

STORIES/TIME

my sister's husband passed away. She was having these awful migraines after he died, so her doctor put her on anti-depressants. Turned out she had brain cancer. The antidepressants may have actually spread the cancer faster. She died last spring. I am now the mother of a soon-to-be one-year-old, and my sister's soon-to-be eighteen-year-old son." She wiped her eyes and laughed, embarrassed. "So, if any of you have any tips on how to raise a teenager . . ."

There were scattered nods. "Don't forget your stone," the director re-minded. Pat waved good-bye with the stone hand. Renny and Liz were staring at me; the story was a glaring lead-in. *I wish I had my hat.*

"That's a hard act to follow!" The next person talked about her teenage son. *Stop listening, and prepare your story. You have to go. Next.*

"I'm Suzy Becker." My speech sounded stiff and shy. "Unh, I had brain surgery. In July. And . . . I am afraid I don't belong here. I'm not the per-son who applied." *Oh, good Christ, someone smother me in a blanket.* I didn't wait for a reminder—I took a stone and sat back down. My story was hanging out there like the *Hindenburg.*

"I didn't have brain surgery," the next woman began softly.

"Can't hear you with the trucks! You're going to have to speak up!" *Thank god it wasn't me—the traffic dies down and you're left shouting your self-revelation.* "I said, I didn't have brain surgery, I'm just shy." She smiled.

"You didn't tell us your name!"

"Sorry. Stacey Collins."

"Can you tell us something about yourself, Stacey?" the director asked. *No story, no rock.* I thought I might get sympathy-sick.

"Like," I interjected, "what sign you are?"

"Aries." People laughed. I got up and held out the basket of stones. The director made a closing comment, and most people skipped out. I left my stone in the grass and went inside to get some punch. *Hey, hello, in case anybody's wondering, I don't have brain cancer! Over here! Just some mild lan-guage problems. I'm going to be fine!*

The people who stayed stuck to the walls of the room and exited abruptly, as if they'd just remembered someplace else they had to be. Stacey caught up with me on my way downstairs. "I wanted to thank you," she said. (People never thank you for those kinds of things.)

"No problem," I said.

"Are you going to be okay?" I wanted to pick her up and hug her. "I think you belong here. I think it's the perfect place for you to heal."

"Thank you, Stacey." *(I said her name, an extra word.)* I knew that she wasn't lying, even if it wasn't the truth.

MEA GULPA

Tim, the speech therapist, had his arm in a sling. He'd had rotator cuff surgery. That made it seem even longer since I'd last seen him.

"Therapy must be easy." I meant convenient, since he worked at a rehab hospital.

"I'm taking it slow. I suppose I'll start to think about therapy at eight weeks, two to three months." When my friend had that surgery, he started the same day. *Maybe that's just for athletes.* "How's it going, Suzy?"

"I need to start speaking more. Telling stories."

"Sounds like a good idea. What's getting in your way?"

"The attention."

"Concentration?"

"People paying attention to me. The mistakes. Having the attention when I make the mistakes." *Just listen to me!* "How do I make less?"

"Practice."

"Sometimes that's worse. The end words come out in the beginning."

"Coarticulation effect. There's not a lot we can do about that." *Then why bother naming it?* "It's still not a bad idea at this stage to think of a story, a cocktail party story"—I must've turned up my nose—"okay, a Bunting story, and try it out on a few friends. I could get a group together, and you could tell your story." *I don't want to tell a pretend group a story. You don't want to get better—is that what you're saying? You haven't done your reading homework either. Maybe I am done. Maybe this is it, as good as I get.*

"Of course, I'm sure there are people you can practice on at home or at the Bunting. You wouldn't have to come all the way in here.

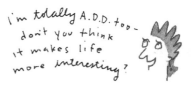

I don't mind coming as long as we DO something!

"How's Harvard treating you?"

"I'm not sure I belong."

A few fellows had approached me since the Grand Circle: "You had brain surgery?! . . . You're doing speech therapy?! Can I get your therapist's number? . . . Well, you must have been *really* funny before, seriously, what were you like?" *I can't answer that, describe me before, like that me is dead. . . .* And when I did describe some of the problems I was having, I got:

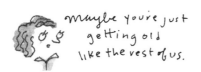

maybe you're just getting old like the rest of us.

I'm totally A.D.D. too— don't you think it makes life more interesting?

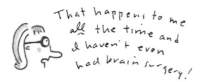

That happens to me all the time and I haven't even had brain surgery!

"I wasn't asked to be part of the writers' group. Could have been a"— *What's the word? Never mind*—"accident. It's just for 'serious' writers. My friend said she'd say something if I really wanted to join—I'm not writing anyway. I don't think I can do a book."

"You can't know until you try."

"I don't know if I'm going to stick with it anyway."

"The fellowship?"

I nodded.

"Could you postpone it, take a few months off and start in January, or, when does the spring semester start?"

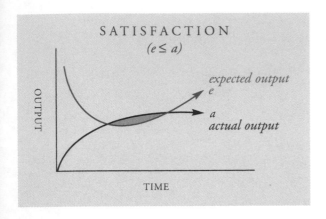

SATISFACTION
$(e \leq a)$

OUTPUT

expected output
e

a
actual output

TIME

I could. *Postponing things doesn't make them easier; sometimes the opposite.* My expectations were getting higher all the time.

"Let me go get you a copy of something, an article I want you to read. It'll actually be good for your reading, too, and then, if there's time, we can discuss it." He handed me a copy of "What Does It Feel Like to Be Brain Damaged?" by a Canadian clinical psychologist who'd been in a car accident. *Five pages, single-spaced at nine minutes each (new reading "speed") = 45 minutes, the rest of the session. Better be worth it.* "It's the only first-person account I've come across in all the medical journals in all the years I've been doing this. It came out in 1985, but I don't think it's dated."

The second paragraph began, "At this point in my recovery, I have a foot in both worlds, for I can remember what it felt like to be completely normal intellectually, and also what it felt like when a loss of function was at its worst." My eyes froze. *I know you were in a coma for a week, and I only had brain surgery, but that is* exactly *how I feel.* "I would read a simple paragraph in the newspaper and by the time I got to the last sentence have no recollection of what the first one was." *Yes.* I slowed down; I wanted to savor each word.

"Having been a highly self-controlled person all my life, I found myself with a hair-trigger temper and labile emotions. It is theorized that this state is due to CNS irritation or else that some part of the brain, which is responsible for 'braking the mental motor,' is dysfunctional." *It was theorized that my state was due to my anxiety, my perfectionism, my inability to manage disappointment. Haven't they seen this article? Why wasn't I told what to expect?*

"Coping is also easier in the milieu that is free from emotional tension, competitiveness, anxiety, and pressure. . . . I find it hard to absorb and retain new information in a meeting with people who are new to me and where there is a constant interchange of ideas and personalities." *I don't care. I'm not giving up this fellowship (I'll never get it again)—they'll have to take it away.*

EVOLUTION OF MY OFFICE

SEPTEMBER

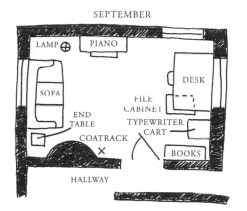

OCTOBER

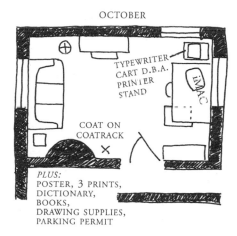

E veryone in my building at the Bunting worked with her door shut. It was so quiet, I could hear Myra when she talked on her phone. In the beginning I left my door half-open, in case someone wanted to visit on the way to or from the bathroom, which I could also hear. Sometimes fellows on the second or third floors met up with one another on the stairway, but I had no reason to go up the stairs. I was lonelier working in the pink gingerbread Victorian than I ever was at home where I saw no one all day. *Maybe I'll take up the piano. Maybe I'll play "Chopsticks" or "The Entertainer" until they have to knock on my door.*

My main focus the first few months was still my recovery. I also hoped to accomplish the following: (1) Get comfortable with the setup—campus, fellows, office, etc.; (2) keep up with *Grist* cartoons; (3) take advantage of downtime and recovery to learn QuarkXpress and Adobe Photoshop.

The first "project" I completed in my office was my mother's seventy-second birthday gift, a scrapbook of the trip to France. I (Suzy Becker, Nonfiction) sat on the floor, surrounded by photos, tickets, receipts, stamps, maps, labels, newspaper clippings, and candy wrappers and assembled the book, spread by spread.

The week after my mother's birthday, I resumed buying the *Globe,* on Thursdays, for the "Calendar" section.

The end of that week, I added another element to my routine. I stopped by the main building for coffee. I said hello to the receptionist on my way downstairs. (The receptionist was an easy hello, a stationary target; a lot of people, I'd noticed, didn't say hello at Harvard, especially in passing.) The kitchen coffeepots were all empty. *Oh, well. Next week.* I pivoted back around to size up the machine. *Same kind as the place where I'd waited tables right out of college.*

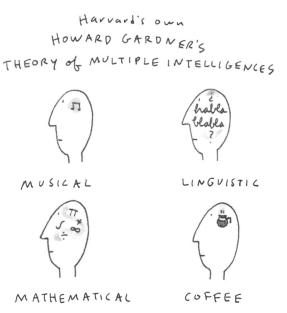

I removed the filter basket, gave it a couple taps, and watched the old filter crumple into the trash can. I emptied a bag of grinds into the new filter and slid the basket back into place; then I poured the water through the screen on top and hit BREW. I held my Styrofoam cup underneath to catch the first stream. When my cup was full, I put the brown (not the orange decaf) pot under, never interrupting the stream, and watched as it hit the glass bottom and began to pool around the edges.

 Mail Message

> Just a reminder about making coffee in the coffeemaker in the main kitchen in building 34. Please take a moment to read the directions above the coffeemaker the next time you make coffee. The directions are on a bright pink sheet of paper and you can't miss them. The directions will instruct you not to add water to the machine. All you have to do is put coffee in the filter, stick an empty pot on the burner and press "brew." The coffeemaker takes water directly from the sink which is then filtered before it makes its way to the coffeemaker. Someone added water to the machine this morning and we had to clean up a flood of coffee from the counter, the floor, and underneath the sink. It also melted the top of the coffeepot so we had to throw it out.

Five days had gone by. I had just finished arranging the mug I brought from home on top of my bookcase. *They had to know it was me!* I was the only fellow in the building Friday morning. I had no choice but to own up. Fess up. Come clean. *Would a coffeepot endowment clear my name? . . . They'll never take another humorist.*

I alternately sat and paced my office, besieged by guilt. A little after three, I saw Natalie, another writer, from my window. She was having a cigarette on the bench outside the kitchen—such a welcome sight!

The cold air did nothing to clear my head as I neared the bench. "Suzy Becker, I didn't realize *you* wrote those little books! Ohmygod, I'm going to embarrass you, I'm such a big fan."

"Y'know the coffeemaker?"

"It was you?"

I nodded. She covered her mouth with her hands, but peals of laughter and snorts escaped through her fingers. I lost my train of thought. I just wanted to make her laugh like that again.

"You're not going to confess, are you?"

Oh, the coffeemaker. "I am, I should—I have to, don't you think?"

"No." She put both hands on top of her cane and pretended to get serious. "The director keeps a spanking stick in her office."

"I'm serious."

"All right—I'll tell you something, but you have to swear not to tell. Last week, I got sick of waiting for that elevator, so I went up the stairs, kind of using the banister to pull myself up and . . . it came off the wall. I stuck it back, but it's not really *on* on."

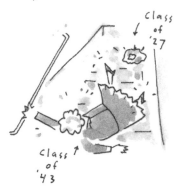

But you've been teaching here five years; they're not going to kick you *out*.

"You can't tell."

I promised.

Dear Fellows,
I am making you lunch in lieu of the optional dinner.
Please sign up and list any dietary restrictions below.
—Natalie

Casey Palmer   No meat, please!
Suzy Becker   Must have dessert.
Gwynne Campbell   nut allergy

Natalie and I became a fixture in the back corner of the colloquium room. We could keep better tabs on our regulars: the woman who thought it was okay to lie down, the woman who talked back to the presenter, the bag woman, the sleepers, nodders, Palm Pilot–updaters, the celebs, unidentified significant others (USOs), the hair fixers, dandruff brushers, and the MacArthur grant nominators.

 Mail Message

> Please refrain from conducting a conversation with your neighbor at any time during the presentation or question-and-answer session. Many of you, guests as well, have engaged in quite lengthy conversations during the presentation. This is disruptive to the speaker and especially disruptive to those seated near you. If you think it is necessary to conduct a conversation during the presentation, please leave the room.

More than a month had gone by, and I still hadn't started my project.

I am so tired (and?) my head hurts. Our first brown bag publishing lunch. We were to say succinctly what our books are about. I don't know (anymore).
I don't know that I can deal with dinner with the fellows tonight. I feel stupid.

It was hard to write a book about whether or not to have a baby when I couldn't even think about having a baby until I was off Neurontin. *What am I doing here? When am I going to be found out?*

I went to my October MRI by myself. Radiology was backed up again, but I had Natalie's memoir, and I was content to read. I read solidly for twenty-five minutes before getting up to call my answering machine and buy a cup of coffee. When I got back, they were ready for me.

It was 6:15 by the time my films were ready. The Brain Tumor Clinic waiting area was empty. At 6:30, Dr. Finn came out to get me himself.

"How *is* everything?"

"I did Ride FAR. I'm at the Bunting." He smiled. "I did ten cartoons." *But don't go thinking I'm all better.* "I'm seventy-five, no, eighty percent."

"Any seizures?" He checked my reflexes and my squeezes. He had me follow his finger with my eyes.

"Can I stop taking the Neurontin?" It wasn't just the baby decision. The drowsiness and thick tongue had worn off. I'd never stopped driving, and the alcohol ban was no big deal—it was the pill thing, the reminder, three times a day, that something was wrong with me.

"It's been three—"

"Four," I corrected him.

"Four months . . . well, the neurologist isn't here." He hesitated. *Please-pleaseplease.* "I don't see why not. Let's have you taper it off over the next two months. That protein mass is pretty well cleared up. I won't need to see you again for a year."

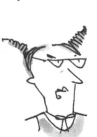

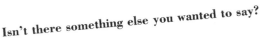

Isn't there something else you wanted to say?

I'll miss you. I wish I could take all this gratitude, respect, and fondness and turn it into sentences.

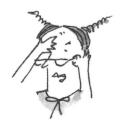

There was something you wanted to ask.

Oh, a stupid, embarrassing question: "Can you check my head?" We both leaned forward. "Is it all right?" I asked. Once every couple of weeks (definitely not more), I forced myself to survey the area. A vertical ridge had developed above the hole, and there still was a hole, the size of my thumbtip.

"Feels pretty good."

But, "I thought I wouldn't have a hole, you put the piece back."

"We did, a piece about so big." He made a rectangle with his thumbs and forefingers. "You've got a hole where the drill went in. I'm afraid you'll always have that."

"And the bump?"

He felt again. "That should settle down."

I had been thinking one of these times, I'd reach up and it would be gone. All smoothed out. Maybe if it were neater, not such a pothole. Or if my brain wasn't under it. A grown-up with a soft spot.

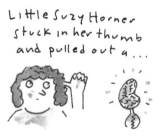

WILLY-NILLY

Please free-write for 10 minutes only about how things are going in general, and specifically with your Bunting Fellowship activities.

I have begun to make friends and feel more like myself. I notice my wit becoming quicker. In small groups, I am beginning to tell longer stories. Sometimes I still worry that someone else should have my place. I am especially hard on myself when I say or do things that make me feel like I am brain damaged.

I am still not settled into a routine. I don't know what level of distraction is normal. I am not used to having so much competition to my work.

My biggest frustration remains when my mouth won't say or my hands won't type or write what I'm thinking.

I really didn't feel like going to speech therapy anymore. I didn't want to drive all the way into town, just to be told to concentrate more or learn to live with it, but I didn't feel *free* enough to write that.

Tim made me read my homework out loud again. When I got to the end he said, "So, you actually have the thought worked out ahead of time, in your head, and you're concentrating, and then—what happens?"

I've told you. "It comes out mixed up—I wish I could concentrate *less.*" I couldn't explain how it felt—like my mind was constantly on a leash. With a choke collar. I'd noticed it when I was doing my cartoons in ink; I used to add last-minute details. Now it took all my concentration to get

my hand to properly trace what was already there, and the
words were hopeless. Every cartoon had at least one
patched-over mistake; most had three or four.

No one can see them!

Tim had a handmade book on his lap.
"I want you to have a look at this story. It's written by a client of mine; her
name's not on it. . . . She's decided she'd like to become a children's book
author. I thought your feedback would be more valuable than mine."

"I'm not an editor," I said, in case this was supposed to be my work-
as-therapy.

It was a story about snowflakes, a be-your-own-snowflake story, actually more of a message than a story—there was no plot. *There's my feedback.*
Something made me reconsider—the handwriting, maybe, reminded me
of Grandma Rosie's. *Who was this woman? Who was she before the accident
in her brain? What kind of feedback is she looking for?* "I can imagine the pictures," was all I said.

"Would you be interested in drawing them?"

Author · Illustrator
MATCHMAKER
for the brain-impaired

"I only do my own." It was the easiest way to phrase the rejection.

He returned the book to her folder and sat back down. "I received
authorization from your insurance company for six more sessions. We'll
have to use the next couple for testing to show we're making progress, but
at the same time, you'd benefit from more therapy. You can stop by the
scheduler's on your way out."

"Oh."

Tell him you're not coming back.

It'll become obvious after a couple of weeks.

I thought of a joke in the car after speech therapy. (I don't usually think of what I'd call "jokes," the stand-alone variety.) Q: What's the difference between the attention span of a cartoonist and someone who's just had brain surgery? A: Wanna see my photographs?

I was brimming-with-joke when I walked into a gallery opening an hour later. My first telling got a mixed reception. It *was* kind of random *and* you'd have to know I'm a cartoonist who's had brain surgery *and,* well, be able to laugh at the latter. I clammed back up.

"Suzy!" It was a woman I had referred to Dr. Finn.

I couldn't remember her name. "How's your daughter?"

"Great, doing really well, but what a scare, huh? *You* know."

"Mm. So she's all okay?"

"They have to keep checking; it was so rare to see that particular tumor in someone her age—she's younger than you—Finn asked her permission to write it up for some medical journal."

I felt an embarrassing twinge of jealousy. "Did you like him?"

"Oh, wonderful, he was wonderful. We'd all but decided to go with the other surgeon—he'd told us that Finn, quote 'shot from the hip' in the O.R.—"

"Wouldn't you want that, if the regular way wasn't working?"

"Once you meet him, there's no one else—thank you so much for the recommendation."

"So, was she—? How was her recovery?"

Really.

"I kept encouraging her to call you, but she was fine with it all. She went back to California the end of the second week. Listen, it was really great to see you." She walked away. *In just a few*

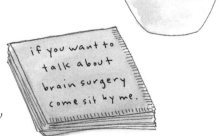

if you want to talk about brain surgery come sit by me.

weeks, I'll be able to have a glass of wine at one of these things. I took an hors d'oeuvre and slipped out.

The
DOUBLE HELIX
of
LOVE

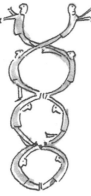

Things with Karen had not improved much since the crash pad argument. One Thursday morning she announced over the phone that she was tired of not being able to meet my expectations. "Clearly, I am not enough, you *need* all your other friends."

My brain was trying to follow and argue at the same time: *I was sitting home alone because her best friend (and her dog) were visiting. I mean, I want the two of you to have time alone—*

"And where *were* your friends all summer? I was the only one who was there for you, but now, now that you're feeling better, I'm always the one that gets dumped on." *I told you to leave me. . . .*

We had fought all these battles before, back in the beginning. This round was bloodier; my weapons, my words were cruder—misfired repeatedly. Scattershot.

I QUIT!

The drive into Cambridge was long and depressing when I wasn't looking forward to seeing Karen.

I sat on my office floor and looked up the word *willy-nilly. Our phone conversation this morning proceeded willy-nilly. Willy-nilly* was right above *Wilson's disease,* the topic of the colloquium just the day before. The synchronicity.

I stared at the photo leaning against my desk lamp. The two of us were smiling, my arms around her neck, in Paris. *I think we're breaking up. Self-correction. I think she wants to break up.* There were times I had been so mad at her, or sad, I had turned this photo over or put it away (not for more than a day). I didn't feel like it.

> **willy-nilly**
> whether desired or not (alteration of will ye, nill ye)

I don't know what I feel. Lost. Those people in the picture are lost. No, their love is lost. They lost that love.

How I once imagined love:

- waking up in someone's arms happy (both of you)
- making love
- showering
- feeling beautiful (both of you)
- making coffee, having coffee in bed
- having breakfast together
- working alone and together
- calling
- writing, drawing, making love-things
- making lunch
- taking walks in new and old places
- visiting
- surprising each other
- having dinner
- not caring about dessert
- wanting to wear dresses
- full heart
- full house
- part of two families
- making new friends (each other's and together)
- playing games
- reading
- reading out loud
- cooking together
- having kids
- traveling in U.S., abroad for weekends, weeks, months
- being proud of each other
- looking out for each other (and each other's dogs)
- wanting each other
- taking each other
- taking each other's hands
- love is the most important thing
- celebrating
- saving things up to tell each other
- making each other laugh
- being happy to see each other

The building doorbell rang. *It's her. She's stopped by to say she's sorry before she goes to Maine.* It was someone visiting Alice upstairs.

Why should I spend another weekend with her? Because I love her. Because I can't bear not to.

Karen didn't want to break up; she wanted to go to couples therapy.

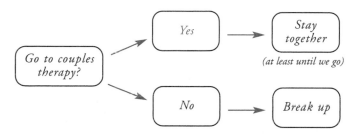

We got a couples therapist through Karen's health plan, someone her therapist had recommended. The woman looked like a younger, Cambridge version of Mrs. Claus. The office was barely big enough for the three of us. On the side table, between Karen's and my chairs, there was a box of tissues and a pyramid-shaped snow scene with pearls that snowed down through a viscous liquid on plastic aquarium plants.

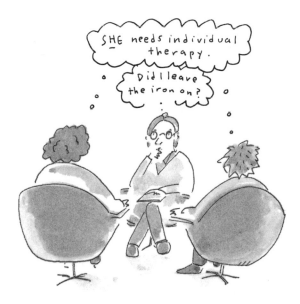

I've forgotten most of the conversations that took place during the handful of sessions we had in there. The gist of it was we went in on the verge of breaking up and came out resolved to stay together, defying the odds. Statistically speaking, most couples enter therapy too late.

The first session began with, "Why are you here?" *To get help, to stay together. Or to break up, if we should—I don't know.* I let Karen answer. She said we were there because we both acknowledged the importance of my friends and family, and we both acknowledged they made Karen feel less important. And because we weren't making love; we weren't living together; the difference in our ages and in when we wanted to go on vacation; our views on skinny-dipping, breakfast, and capitalism. Karen laughed, like it was funny. I cried; my lability embarrassed me.

At the second session, the therapist thought it would be helpful to both of us and our relationship if I answered the question, "What is the difference between a friend and a lover?"

Isn't it obvious? "My lover is the first person I want to talk to when I wake up; the last person I want to talk to before I fall asleep. The person I want to fall asleep next to. The person I want to tell the best news or the worst news." *Isn't the question really, "What would make Karen feel like my lover?"* "My emergency contact—"

"The difference?"

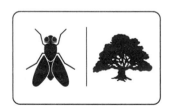

Besides what I just said? I couldn't think. "The way you spend your time. I organize my days around being with Karen." *Not with Bruce or anybody else.* My head was filling up with viscous liquid. "I don't know. Ask my friends. They all know the difference. And my family. Everyone knows that Karen is the most important—"

"Suzy," the therapist interrupted, "where's your heart? I don't hear your heart. I think that's what Karen needs to hear. Some abandon."

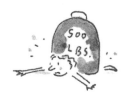

I broke down. *Where* is *my heart? My abandon?* "I don't know."

I believed love was the most important thing *and* my lover didn't feel loved: I was a failure at the most important thing. I didn't feel loved, either, but I would have, I was sure, if she did. I felt pressure to make love. I felt pressure to get better so we could get back to the way we were before it all happened.

but you're a success at so many things like, like

There was something else I couldn't articulate then. There is no separation of head and heart; it's a romantic notion, make-believe—like Santa Claus or the tooth fairy. Brain surgery had ruined it for me; I could never go back to believing. My heart was in my brain (part of the 20 percent that wasn't back), which explained why I still didn't feel like *me*.

At the time, all I had was a sense, a worry that I would never find my heart and my abandon with Karen. *It's too hard.*

I never said the words; something stopped me. Something inside me insisted on her. Her hands. Her eyes. Her voice. She had seen me through all this.

Our relationship was like being at Harvard. It took everything I had when I was at my best. That's where I wanted to be, again. I wasn't going to quit.

Nothing's *too* hard, if it's what you want. It just *is*.

There was my heart.

KINDRED SPIRITS

By the second week in November, I was feeling 85 percent. I met my agent for lunch; I was hoping a conversation about the book project would give me enough clarity or motivation to begin.

"Why don't you work on your I Can Read book until you're ready to start the other?"

The editor had never returned the manuscript. "Can you call Robert and—?"

"I think you should have a conversation with him. When was the last time you two talked?"

"But he doesn't know about my brain."

"No reason why he should. You can call him."

I called him the next day. The pay phone was in the front hall closet of the main building. Another fellow walked in on me (to use the phone, no one used it as a closet), and I took advantage of the interruption to end the conversation. My manuscript would be returned to me by Thanksgiving.

I used the next two weeks (and the $180 I had left in my Ride FAR gift certificate) to plan a Thanksgiving brunch at the bakery the Sunday before the actual holiday. I invited everyone on the long thank-you list I had kept in the back of my desk calendar.

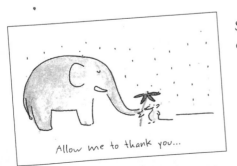

Allow me to thank you...

Partway through the brunch, one of the guests who'd traveled from Maine asked if I was going to say anything. *As in to everyone, all at once?* "Do you think I need to?"

"I think that people will expect you to say *some*thing," she answered.

Old me might have. New me couldn't without any preparation. I decided it was enough to host a gathering. I looked around the room and felt grateful, not resentful. *That was progress.*

T hanksgiving dinner, my sisters, my mother, Jonathan, Karen, and I were gathered around Robin's kitchen table. She revived the things-to-be-thankful-for alternative-grace tradition, which was scuttled in 1992 when my mother interrupted my thanks—that my best friend could join us—to say that *she* used to be my best friend. This year, everybody was thankful that I was healthy.

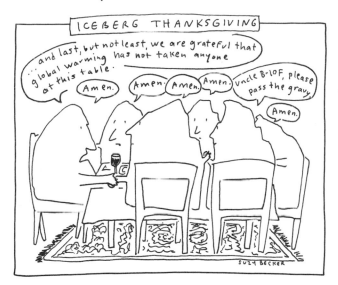

I took my last dose of Neurontin on November 30 and put the remaining three pills in with the box of worry dolls I kept on my desk at the Bunting. It had been seven months since the grand mal seizure, five since the surgery. On December 1, the first day I could drive legally and drink, Karen and I celebrated our sixteen-month anniversary with mojitos.

My energy level was almost back to normal. The season stimulated my impulse to give, and I allowed myself to get swept up in preparations. Christmas would be, as it had been for the last ten years, at my place.

Mid-December, there was a small wrench thrown in the works. Karen complained she'd been feeling something in the back of her throat, and her doctor ordered a barium swallow on a Friday afternoon. I stood by the technician and watched the monitor like a hawk. Only, it turns out, I was no hawk. I couldn't begin to fathom what I was looking at. They had her swallow more and more, she was on her second bottle of barium, and the images looked identical. "Is that something?" I asked when the technician froze a frame and started typing.

"Which?" the technician asked.

"On the screen. Is it okay?" She didn't answer. "What are you typing?"

"I'm labeling the image." Karen would have gotten more out of her.

They finished the test. "I can get dressed, but we're supposed to wait, make sure they don't need any more images." I followed Karen back to the dressing room. We had just found seats in the waiting area when the technician appeared in the doorway. "They're good."

"You read them?" I could hear the relief in Karen's voice.

I took her hand. "She means she has enough pictures," I said quietly.

"The doctor will read them and give you a call next week."

"Monday," Karen said.

"If that's what she said. Good luck!"

"Good luck?" Karen turned toward me. "She saw something, why else would she wish me good luck?"

"They always say that, 'Good luck,' like, 'I hope the doctor doesn't see anything.'"

"Did you see anything?"

"I couldn't tell—I'm sorry."

We spent the weekend alone; Karen didn't want to see anyone. We went to a concert, drove around looking at Christmas lights. When we were in bed on Saturday night, Karen said, "I really don't want to die." I held her. I was *so* sure she wasn't going to, it made me nervous. *The perfect setup: I (the younger one) have a scare. Then, just when we think we're on the other side, maybe we're feeling a little arrogant—BLAM! It's her.*

I pressed my ear up against the back of the receiver after she'd dialed the doctor on Monday morning, but she walked into the bathroom and closed the door once her doctor picked up. The door opened. "Looks like I'm going to be around to torment you a few more years!"

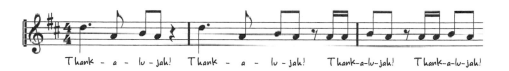

Thank - a - lu - jah!   Thank - a - lu - jah!   Thank-a-lu-jah!   Thank-a-lu-jah!

"Well, I better start your Christmas shopping."

"Suz?" *You love me? Thanks for being there?* "I *really* need a vacation."

Either I was on one or I didn't qualify for one. It was hard enough not making money, living off my savings, but—"Hello? Are you there? Suz, we haven't had a vacation . . . Paris with your brain tumor doesn't count. I'm used to going away for Christmas and New Year's, and I'm willing to compromise, but—"

"After my colloquium?" *Colloquium! I said it!*

"The end of March? That's too far away."

vacation a period of time devoted to pleasure, rest, or relaxation esp. one with pay, from Latin *vacatio*, freedom from occupation

We planned a trip to Placencia, Belize, in late January. The deal was, I had to begin my Bunting baby-decision-brain-surgery-whatever-it-was-going-to-be book project and work on it every day while we were there.

The first morning, Karen went out and left me alone at the small desk in our room. I set out a brand-new pad of yellow graph paper, book writing paper. (I write my first drafts longhand so I can switch back and forth between writing and drawing.) I opened my Bunting notebook and set it beside the yellow pad. Then I began writing in the notebook, as if the momentum might carry my hand across the divide onto the yellow pad.

The second morning, when I still hadn't cracked the yellow pad, I re-sorted to my old carrot-and-stick: *This is the hardest part, the beginning; once you have the beginning, the middle is easy, and the end will write itself. . . .*

The third morning: *Doing nothing is doing something. All part of the process. Eventually you will become so fed up with doing nothing, you will have to do something.*

On the fifth day of vacation, we moved up the peninsula to a grass ca-bana on the beach. I'd discovered the place on a rented mountain bike. Chuck, the owner, had offered to drive us out from town, as long as the soap patch in his gas tank held. "In the U.S., you drive on the right. In the U.K., they drive on the left. In Belize, we drive on the best side," he joked as we bounced into the driveway and he stopped short to avoid crushing a column of fire ants. "Don't want to kill these little guys, they eat up all in-sects. Look, they got a scorpion! Big, fat one." Karen and I traded faces.

I began this book at Chuck's place that afternoon. We fell asleep before ten that first night, and after midnight, I was jolted out of a deep sleep. Something landed on my forehead. I kept my head perfectly still and nudged Karen. She turned over without waking up; I nudged her a second time, "Wake up! I have a squid on my head!"

"Huh?"

"I have a *squid* on my head!"

"I don't understand what you're saying."

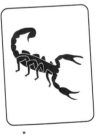

What's not to understand? Get it off my head before it stings me! I repeated it a third time; that time I heard myself. *Not a squid.* "A— the thing the ants had."

"A scorpion?"

"*Yes!* On my head!"

She turned on the light and calmly reached for my head. "It's a caterpillar."

"Vacation hasn't helped my speech."

"You're *too* relaxed. I think somewhere in between Harvard and here." We draped the mosquito netting over the bed and went back to sleep.

After making Karen do all the talking—all the phone calls, questions, and menu-ordering—the whole trip, I talked to the woman sitting next to us on the plane from Belize to Houston, four hours. I didn't realize how much I missed talking to strangers. She was on her way home to England after visiting her younger sister, who moved to Belize during World War II. She still missed her terribly after all this time. She had hoped her daughter-in-law would be a kindred spirit, but no such luck, and her other son wasn't married. She raised her eyebrows. "He's older than you."

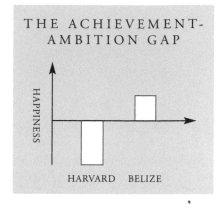

THE ACHIEVEMENT-AMBITION GAP

HAPPINESS

HARVARD   BELIZE

I told her my little sister and I were kindred spirits. She said her sister was trying to persuade her to move out of her little village to the city, where she wouldn't have to drive. "I'm not ready yet, and it shouldn't matter what my sister or anybody else thinks . . . but it does. People say all kinds of things about my son." I figured it had to do with his being unmarried.

I asked if he seemed lonely. No, he had lots of friends. Lovely friends who not only love him, they treat her like a queen.

Then, I agreed, it shouldn't matter. We were quiet for a few minutes. "What *do* they say? Do they say he's"—*Would she understand "gay"?* — "a homosexual?"

"They say Philip's gay. I don't know if he is or not. He's never said, and I've never asked him. But, if he was"—she turned to look at me—"I'd put my arms around him and say, 'That's okay, Philip, I love you.'"

You have to say something. "Well, I think you should tell him that. Exactly that." And I didn't stop there. I told her Karen and I were lovers and how my parents had only recently started telling people I was gay. She told me all about Philip and his roommate.

As we landed, I had one hand on Karen's leg, and the woman held on to the other. She said, "You and I are kindred spirits. Don't you think we were meant to sit next to each other?"

If I say yes, does that mean everything up until now was meant to be, too?

ERMA BOMBECK, ROLL OVER!

Grand Circle Number Two, the progress report, took place while we were in Belize. It was grim by all accounts. The academic job market was tight, and there were no stones for the taking. I was glad I missed it. The anxiety around the Bunting was contagious; I'd caught myself worrying I didn't have a job and had to remind myself I wasn't looking.

It wasn't a good place to rest, it was relentless—I was constantly comparing myself with the other fellows. But it was a good place to heal. I think the striving was better for my recovery than working alone.

I was relentless, always keeping track of myself: my self as a percentage of my old self.

My Language Problems

Location	Writing/Speech	This	Not That
Karen's	S	dinner	breakfast
Office	W	chicken	kitchen
Office	W	daughters	doctors
Office	W	loose	soon
Meeting	S	minutes	months
Bakery	S	sticky bone	sticky bun
Restaurant	S	Chapsticks	chop sticks
Home	S	Polaroid	polar bear

Like Renny said, Harvard is intimidating. And, these kinds of things happen to everybody. Little lapses. *But which are the real lapses: the lapses or the times in between?*

Mild TBI Moments

9/\3   Getting keys. Creativewriting/nonfiction incident.

9/30   Oral invite to Harvard/Radcliffe merger at \2.
         I asked, "Is that noon or midnight?"

\0/8   Coffeemaker.

\0/28   Car towed with Mister on street-cleaning day.

\\/\8   Patricia Hampl, MacArthur Fellow book signing.
         She asked the spelling of my name for inscription.
         P: Why'd you pick that one?
         S: My mother liked the "z."
         P: I meant that book.

\\/25   Put overnight bag behind car to remember to pack.
         Ran over overnight bag.

\\/26   Shoveled snow off hood of car with metal shovel.
         Scratched hood.

To me, they were all reminders my head had been opened up; my brain was exposed to the air. My scar was showing. I was brain injured, brain damaged.

brain·dead · one 🗡 blade short of a sharp edge · a 🍔 burger short of a barbecue · not playing with a full 🎴 deck · not the full 🍾 bottle · not the sharpest ✏ pencil in the box · not the sharpest 🪚 tool in the shed · not a rocket 🚀 scientist, and most definitely 𝓕 not a brain surgeon.

Or maybe I *was* just getting older, like everybody else. The self, the sense of mastery and possibility I was trying to get back, belonged in my twenties. Brain surgery reset my clock, ahead, somewhere between age forty and fifty. *I better get used to it; be more patient with myself; gracefully accept my losses. It was going to get worse, not better.*

When I was in high school, I used to wish Grandma Belle wouldn't be so hard on herself. Now I knew what she must have been thinking: *You cut yourself some slack, and know what you end up with? A lot of slack.*

The second semester, I decided to try some slack; I quit keeping tabs— no more records of any kind (except when I said "Brain Jody" instead of "Jane Brody"; I wouldn't want to forget that). I audited a class taught by the comparative religion professor Renny had recommended, and I signed up for the graduate student discussion section.

Alternative Therapies

1. Discussion section for course (modified book group)

2. Catalog (numbers/speech) therapy: Attempt to place catalog order. (Must dial number, say catalog no., source code no., item no., and credit card no. with exp. date correctly the first time or order is invalid.)

3. Chicken (writing/drawing) therapy: Every day you don't work, you have to draw an exotic chicken.

I had to get serious about my work. My colloquium was eight weeks away. Once I decided to begin with a reading (and slides) from *Macro Mary* (the application writing sample Renny loved), I was less nervous about having enough material. I just needed twenty minutes, twenty new pages. *Twenty* good *pages. And slides.*

I had eight weeks. *Seven weeks. One week to rehearse.* It still sounded as if it might be doable.

The middle of the second week of February, I drove out to Northampton to go to a concert with Meredith. Things were better between us, but not back to the way they used to be. The band came on late, which gave us an extra hour to talk. After the second song, we looked at each other through the smoke. It was a school night: "Last song?"

We stood outside the club in the clear, cold February air. "I wish you were staying at my place," she said, "but I know Robin wants to see you— I'm glad, I mean, it's good you two have become close."

The snow was seeping up through my soles. "I love you, Mer."

"I miss you," she said. "I don't want to have to wait until we're routing Ride FAR 7 to spend time together—do you ever think like that?"

"We won't."

The next morning, I lay awake with Mister on Robin's couch just looking around, waiting for Robin to come out of her room. Her apartment is like a big refrigerator door. There are paintings on the walls, paintings on the floors, pieces she got in trade for her jewelry, pieces she got out of the trash. There are letters, photographs, old cards, postcards, every watch she's ever owned—and you want to look at all of it. I picked out the things I had contributed over the years: a dragon drawn with new markers when I was twelve, an *All I Need to Know* poster, six valentines. I got up to examine a photograph I'd sewn with copper wire onto a screen, as if it were someone else's work. The matchbox with a red heart made of match tips. My first oil-stick landscape, on vellum. *I used to be so . . . clever. And so generous. I didn't used to be so . . . afraid.*

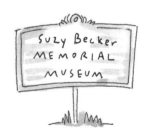

I lay back down. *You've felt this way before. Felt like I'm going down the drain? Thanks. Is that supposed to be some sort of consolation?*

On the drive back home, it hit me: *I have felt this way before.* This *is anxiety, good ole, plain ole, ole-fashioned anxiety!* I just hadn't recognized it coming from this angle.

I know how to get back from here!

I was anxious about my colloquium. *Ha! Nothing brain damaged about that!* When I got home, I moved an old wooden desk out of the barn into my bedroom and sat it at an angle under the eaves. Empty, no distractions. Just a lamp and the yellow pad. And comforting—the eaves and my bed close by.

Saturday through Tuesday, I wrote in my bedroom. Wednesday through Friday, I wrote at the Bunting.

By then I had made a couple of friends in the building. Liz was on the third floor. Alice was at the top of the stairs. I would run up and flop down in her armchair for a five-minute break. (I was less adept at managing breaks in my own office.)

Break Management

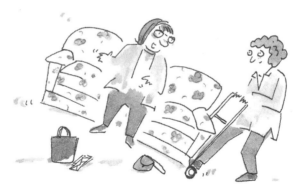

Pat, across the hall, was a chaired professor and department head at Barnard. She was friendly, always busy (from what I could see through four inches of open door), and dauntingly poised. We swapped coffee runs.

Just for practice!

The day after her colloquium, one month before mine, I left a box of chocolates and a congratulations card outside her door. I was in my office, preparing for interviews with publishers at "Publications Day." I was actually lying on my floor trying to come up with a new title for my book, since it no longer had anything to do with a baby. It was about my brain surgery.

> PUBLICATIONS DAY INTERVIEWER: I'm not arguing with the fact you had brain surgery; I'm just not sure there's a book in it. A lot of what you've just finished describing happens to me and *[chuckle]* I haven't even had brain surgery.

Then what do I say? What do I usually say?

> ME: Well, what's *your* excuse? *[chuckle]*

There was a knock at the door. I stopped chuckling and sat up. "Come in!" It was Pat.

"Looks like you're having fun. What were you laughing at?"

Something that I wouldn't think was funny if my sister had died of brain cancer. "I thought of a new title."

"Let's hear it!"

"I don't really think it works." She made me say it. "*I Had Brain Surgery, What's Your Excuse?*" She burst out laughing.

"That's great! What's it for?"

"My book project."

"Wait, I thought you were working on a pregnancy thing—you didn't really have brain surgery, did you?" I'd forgotten she left the Grand Circle before my turn.

"I did."

"My sister—"

"I know, I mean, what you said at the beginning of the year. I'm sorry. I don't, I can't bear to think about losing one of my sisters. I keep thinking it's weird how our offices ended up next door to each other. Makes it hard to forget how lucky I am. I wonder all the time if I would've been able to write this book, if I would've thought any of it was funny, if things had turned out differently."

She sat down on the floor. "Of course you would have. Maybe not the book, but you're the same person—if you use humor to deal with things, that's how you'd deal with them. My sister was hilarious. Sometimes it was kind of a black humor." Pat asked about my prognosis, and I told her what Dr. Finn had said. Dr. Finn had helped her manage her sister's case in Philadelphia; now, she and her husband host families for Boston's Brain Tumor Society.

Pat let herself out. "I don't want to take any more of your time. I just wanted to thank you for the chocolates; that was very sweet. I can't wait for your colloquium, it's going to be great!"

Karen enabled me to continue my lifelong avoidance of AV equipment by making all my colloquium slides and offering to run the two projectors. I booked five hours of rehearsal time, the Sunday and Tuesday before the Wednesday colloquium so we could get our timing down.

Sunday's rehearsal was tense. It took three hours to get through the presentation one time. In order for the slides to work in counterpoint to the text, we had to pin down exactly when each slide came up, and went down. Most of the time, my back was to the slides, unless I needed to emphasize or explain something. "Bear with me while I try PowerPoint," I read, the lead-in to my putting on a big red foam finger.

I couldn't make out Karen's expression, the way the projectors were casting shadows across her face. I stepped to the side of the podium. "Does that work, or should I just skip it?"

"Yes, it works, keep going."

"It would help if you laughed. Maybe I should cut it."

"Sweetie, I have two projectors going."

I highlighted the parts of the text that gave me problems, the way Tim had suggested—dates, names, polysyllabic words, phrases I either stumbled over or left out repeatedly—so I could go over them later, alone.

When I finished, Karen dimmed the projectors and lay down on the floor. "I am so tired." She was squinting.

"Whabut about me?" It sounded like *Zoom!* talk.

"What about you, Suz?"

"I know, sorry. Never mind—"

"Suz, let me finish. Your colloquium will be wonderful. Everybody is going to love it. But right now, my back is killing me. I have to find something to sit on for Wednesday. I can't stand that long: I'm too old."

"I'm sorry." I lay down on the floor beside her and turned her face toward me. "Thank you. It *is* about you, too, you know—"

"Suz, it's your story. I'm happy to help you—"

"Part of the story is about how much I love you. Part of it is our story." She wasn't convinced.

The morning of my colloquium, my dad called to wish me good luck. My mother called to see if there was anything she could do.

Robin and I had lunch; then I did one final read-through. She picked up the pages as I turned them over and read them. "Suz, I didn't realize it was so personal." *Too personal? Too late.* "I didn't mean too personal. I'm glad Meredith decided to come."

I wouldn't know if I was glad until it was all over. I put Cathy Freed's good-luck penny in my pants pocket, and we drove to the Bunting. "Mommy's in the parking lot," Robin said as we were getting out of the car.

"You have her parking pass, and the elevator is to the right of the stairs—"

"She's going to be upset if she sees you walking in without saying hello first." I headed for the parking lot. Meredith was just getting out of her car. My mother held out a bunch of roses. "These are for you, Suzy."

"Better wait and see how I do . . ." I kissed her and looked up to find Meredith. My dad was standing there, as unexpected and as welcome as that first night in the hospital.

He smoothed the back of my hair before resting his hand on my shoulder. "I couldn't miss this."

All of a sudden, I felt nervous. Laura was walking toward us. My agent was sitting by the door. "I'd better go." I ducked in the side entrance and took the elevator up to the colloquium room. It was 3:30; there were a few people—strangers—already seated, reading. I filled my Stone Cold Steve Austin water bottle and set it inside the podium. The foam finger was hidden down below. I opened my folder and laid a watch down beside it. I had never been so prepared.

Karen arrived at 3:50, straight from a meeting. Harried and apologetic. "I've got to find a stool."

"Found it. And I put a glass of water back there for you."

"Have they touched the projectors?"

"All set," I said, and grabbed her forearms. "I'm nervous."

"Wow, you've got a roomful! Good luck, sweetie." She squeezed my hands and let go. "You better go sit down."

I took my seat up front, next to Renny. "I hope you ordered enough dinner." She smiled. "You ready?"

"Mm." I nodded. *Ready as I'll ever be.* She stood up. *Wait! I didn't mean ready this second!*

She began her introduction. I remember one word—*fey*—the word my publisher used in his recommendation to describe my humor. I had had to look it up, pre–brain surgery.

When Renny finished, I stood, took a deep breath, and walked to the podium. "I want to begin by thanking Renny for that wonderful introduction"—I was the twenty-fifth fellow to begin the same way—"although, it's a little awkward to point out, she actually overlooked a couple of my accomplishments."

Slide 1　　　　　　　　　　　　　　　　*Slide 2*

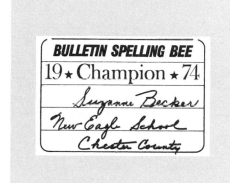

I had them! I read *Macro Mary* and what were then the first twenty pages of this book, ending with the result of the CAT scan, the first report of the mass in my head. Big sip of Stone Cold water. "It's 5:15." Karen flashed a slide of pizza. "I have time to take a few questions." I put the foam finger back on to call on people.

No hands. *The material was too accessible. Worse, too personal.* Bruce's mother raised her hand. "Will we get to see more of Augusta?"

"Definitely!" *With answers like that, you're sure to get more questions.*

Another hand—this time someone I didn't recognize. "Was your sense of humor always this weird, or do you think it was the brain surgery?" She got big laughs.

"Thanks, I mean, am I supposed to answer that? There are a lot of people in the room who've known me for a long time and could probably answer it better. Maybe we should all go downstairs and get some pizza—oh, wait!" I caught myself, *ingrate!* "I need to thank all the people—the Bunting staff and the fellows who helped me with my presentation." I had a list. "My friends Laura and Bruce, my agent Edite, and last, most of all, my partner, the lovely projectionist, Karen Simpson."

People filed forward; I stepped in front of the podium to greet the woman who had asked the last question. "Congratulations, Suzy!" She told me her name. "I've had two craniotomies and a bleeding aneurysm, and I wanted to thank you, your humor is so necessary." She hugged me.

The P.O.ed (Possibly Offended)

~~Pat~~	Dr. Thompson, Laura
Buddha	Mother, father, sisters, brother
Dr. Finn	Karen
~~Other patients~~	Therapist
Harvard	Straight people, gay people

My parents were still in their seats. My dad stood. "Wonderful, Suetta."

"*Verklempt.*" Meredith elbowed my dad.

"I'm going to tell my friend Rosemary she can stop praying." My mother hugged me.

"It was hard for me to hear about those seizures. You never told me about any of that," my dad said.

"Or your mother," my mother chimed in.

"I never told anybody."

My dad fiddled with his shirt button. "I don't like to think about you going through that alone."

"You don't have to." I looked back in Karen's direction; she had a crowd around her. I walked back and broke in. "I have to thank my girlfriend." I gave her a kiss on the cheek. "You know the flower shop we walk by in the morning?"

"The one with the sunflowers?"

"They're fake." I'd gone to get her some.

"And we thought we were awake." She laughed. I suddenly felt so empty-handed.

Downstairs, Renny did the traditional toast. More than forty people stayed for dinner. And stayed and stayed. Karen started cleaning up around the people, and they still stayed, at which point, I announced that they should feel free to stay as long as they liked, but we were going. And, as no one even looked up during my announcement, we walked out.

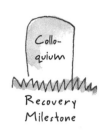

Collo-
quium

Recovery
Milestone

My brown-bag lunch was the next day. When Renny turned the conversation over to me, I was supposed to frame the feedback I was about to receive. "I'm interested in"—*What's the bigger word for* other? *Shit*—"other ways of presenting information. Charts, graphs, diagrams, tables, theorems—things I might be able to use from your field."

The fellow sitting to my right responded first. "I had a question. Is *I Had Brain Surgery, What's Your Excuse?* the title? I guess I'm asking if you're committed to using it; I liked *Fertile Mind* so much better."

"I want to save that title for that book."

"It just sounds so Dave Barry or something." Harvard translation: 𝔜𝔬𝔲 commercial slut.

"No, no," someone else volunteered, "whatscrname, Erma Bombeck." Harvard translation: 𝔜𝔬𝔲 commercial unfeminist slut.

I drank some water. I had not touched my lunch, and I noticed I was crouching in my chair, both feet on the seat.

Pat asked, "Your relationship with Karen is so strong now. How did the whole experience change it? Or did it?"

"Well, my speech (you know) was im—affected by the surgery, so it went from being a verbal relationship between two very independent people to my being nonverbal and dependent. I really believed for a while that Karen should leave me; I wasn't able to be anybody's partner. As I got, still am getting better, more independent, we've had a lot of the same fights we had in the beginning.

"I wish, we both wished we could go back to the honeymoon stage—we hadn't been together that long when the whole thing started. It's just within the last month we realized, it sounds obvious when you say it, but, you can't go back. It's sad, but helpful, to me anyway, because, the whole time, I've been trying to get my 'self' back . . . and it's the same thing.

"We've been together almost two years now, feels like ten—and that feels good, more solid than the honeymoon stage."

Karen and I were lying in bed after *ER*. We replayed the colloquium events start to finish. I was euphoric. Exhausted. Relieved. I was going to be able to have my career back. I never would have attributed so much of my "self" to work (I thought only workaholics did), but now that I knew I could work again, I felt like my old self was back. And it was strange *and, comparatively-religiously speaking, un-Buddhist* to recognize how important my faith in a future was to my present self.

I fell asleep with Karen's arm curled around my waist and woke up the same way ten hours later. I hadn't slept late in months. *Nine?* And I hadn't awakened with nothing to prove, nothing making me not want to get out of bed in just as long.

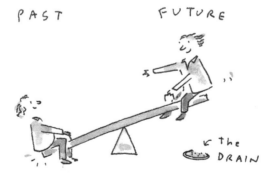

The LAST CHAPTER

not final

Sometime in May or June, I stopped thinking of myself as a person who had just had brain surgery. I happened to be seated next to the head of surgery at Brigham and Women's Hospital at a dinner, and I asked him about the phenomenon. "Do you know how long people identify as"—I didn't exactly know what to call us—"surgery survivors? Like David Letterman and the videotape of his bypass. Can you predict, will that go away by November?"

There weren't any studies he was aware of. "It's probably like grief, varies from person to person."

That was really the only noticeable progress I'd made in the months since the colloquium. I suppose I could have gone back for testing. I had my own tests; I wasn't as quick as Meredith or some of the fellows, but I was comfortable, holding my own most of the time. I still had six months left in my recovery window.

Lasting effects

Concentration—everything more effortful	Short-term memory
	Mild attention deficit
Less spontaneity	Confidence down
Headaches, balance when tired	Quickness down
Word retrieval	Feelings of mortality
Spelling	Oral miscues
Sequencing—writing, speech	Reading out loud
Proofreading	Handwriting

Karen was guarding our spot on the beach in her flag shirt while Bruce and I stood in line at a burger shack. He handed me a box of sparklers and a card. "I gave Bill a card on the one-year anniversary of his surgery, and he said I remembered the date better than he did."

"Fourth of July, well, *that* one's too hard to forget." We laughed.

The three of us watched the fireworks explode over the harbor. "Not bad for a little town," Karen said.

Much better than last year. But there was still room for improvement. "Boston next year?"

STATUS OF PROMISES

	KEPT	BROKEN
FORGET CONVERSATION ABOUT WILL		•
VOLUNTEER AT HOSPITAL		•
NOT TO COMPLAIN ABOUT LITTLE THINGS		•
NOT TO BE A POLLYANNA	•	
PAINT		•
REST		•
LEARN PHOTOSHOP AND QUARK		•
BOSTON FIREWORKS		•

Four months later (November 2000)

Karen and I walked by the ultrasound department on our way to radiology. "The hallway is so much brighter than I remembered," I said. My memory squirmed in the light. I didn't trust myself. *Which self?* My perspective kept shifting with time.

"It was closed when we were here, remember—the Fourth of July, the director had to come in?" *Phew.* I remembered.

It had been a year since I'd been in the hospital.

After we sat down in the waiting room, twelve months' worth of doubts crawled out—every headache, twinge, and tremor.

The nurse had me put a johnny on and then led me to a chair. "Have a seat and roll up your sleeve. Are you right- or left-handed?"

"I'm getting an MRI."

"A dye-enhanced MRI."

"Are you sure? I always get the regular, can you check? I'm allergic to shellfish, iodine—"

"This isn't iodine; it's completely nonallergenic." She missed the vein; I'd rattled her. "I'm going to get someone else to take care of you. We haven't had a good start."

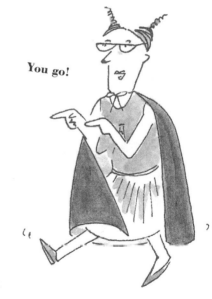

You go!

After the MRI, I made notes about the ultrasound department, the MRI, and the woman next to me (who was reading about the healing power of celery seed) while we waited for my films. Karen was working on an historical booklet of Boston's waterfront. After half an hour, I went to check on the status of my films, and Karen went upstairs to get coffee.

She handed me a latte and dropped a little bag in my lap. "I went to the gift shop." It was a Mister finger puppet. "He wishes he could be here."

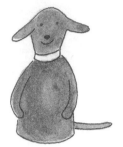

I WISH WE WERE ALL IN THE WOODS ROLLING IN SoMETHING smelly.

Dr. Finn looked at the films. "You look perfect." (He meant the films.) "How do you feel?"

"I'll pass on the lobotomy."

"Do you remember what you said one of the first times I asked? You said you'd lost your impulse. I was ready to hang up my gloves." *Me, my big mouth, and my little problems.* I felt bad.

"What about this 'potential for neoplasm'?" Karen was referring to the diagnostic report.

"Scar tissue." *New scar tissue from removing the old scar tissue?* "Do *you* have any questions?" he asked me.

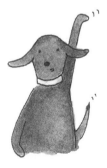

I HAVE A QUESTION— was the surgery *really* necessary?

Isn't it a little late to ask? "What if I never had the surgery?"

"You would have continued to have seizures, and they were getting worse, weren't they? As they worsened, they may have impacted your speech, from what we know now about the way your brain is organized."

It was a satisfactory answer, but the question keeps kicking around.

"I don't need to see you for three years."

"Sounds like a clean bill of health to me, Suz." Karen put her arm around me.

We shook hands good-bye and left Dr. Finn's office. *Three years!* I wondered if he'd remember me.

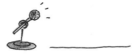

TERRY GROSS: Is that the point at which you considered yourself fully recovered?

ME: It's the point when I started calling myself, reset myself to 100 percent. The maturational benefits of the life experience zero out the lasting deficits. I'm still recovering; it takes a long time for the confidence to come back.

TG: You had a pretty remarkable recovery.

ME: The brain is remarkable. After Ride FAR, I said to my dad, this kind of thing teaches you you're both stronger and more vulnerable than you ever knew. He had a massive heart attack when he was forty-two, and he said you'd be surprised how fast you forget the strength part when you're faced with the next thing.

> To be seriously ill in your forties toughens you for a long life.
>
> —G. B. SHAW

TG: You mentioned the maturational aspects.

Yes, and it felt like a heap of cow crap when it came out of my mouth.

TG: What did you get out of the experience?

ME: I'll probably know better in ten years. . . .

TG: Not as fresh . . .

ME: I regained, in some ways found, an appreciation for a lot of things. Cartooning was a big one. I never realized how finding the humor in things, circumstances, gives me a feeling of power over them. . . . Just looking for humor—I'm lucky that's what I do.

I'm much closer to my older sister, Robin. And to Karen. After someone sees you through something like this . . .

I like to think I got better at accepting help. I know I learned a lot about offering it. Maybe I'm a little less of a perfectionist.

I learned a ton about the brain. I read a lot, but the experience . . . everything is—I don't know if I'll say *run*—processed by your brain.

Oh, and I'm seizure-free. It's been so long, I practically forgot what they were like.

TG: And you got a book. Was writing this book therapeutic?

ME: Yes. And no. When I started what I thought was this book, it was like a friend I could tell everything who never got sick of listening. It was so important, urgent, to remember, record every last detail. Once I wrote it down, I didn't have to carry it around in my head anymore. . . . . After my colloquium, I was really ready to move on; reliving it was like that movie *Groundhog Day.* I had a lot of nightmares. But looking back on it now, I don't know what else I would have done during that time. It was my own work as therapy, speech-occupational therapy.

TG: You must feel good now that it's done.

ME: Really good.

Except the part of me that thinks it would have been better, written better, if I had never had brain surgery.

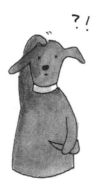

READERS GUIDE
QUESTIONS FOR DISCUSSION

1. *I Had Brain Surgery, What's Your Excuse?* is an illustrated memoir—a new and certainly unusual form. What role do the graphics play in the narrative? Are they strictly illustrative, or do they move the story along? Did they help or hinder your reading experience?

2. What do you think of the title of the book? Do you find it funny? Engaging? Or too in-your-face?

3. Becker says, "Finding the humor in things gives me a feeling of power over them." What do you think she means? Is humor a coping mechanism or a way of avoiding the truth, a way of keeping others at arm's length? Did Becker's sense of humor make you feel closer to her? In general, are you made uneasy when a serious subject is treated in a humorous way? Is nothing sacred . . . not even brain surgery?

4. The author clearly has a vivid interior life; after all, how many of us imagine radio interviews with NPR hosts? Is this a mark of creativity? How does your own inner life compare? Were you able to relate to the voices in Becker's head, who then became characters in the book? Did you have a favorite?

5. Suzy Becker's brain surgery was her first real experience with the medical system. Do you think her experiences—as well as her reactions to them—are typical? Why do doctors inspire such strong emotional responses (awe and anger being just two) in so many of us?

6. When Becker's first physician told her that her seizures were probably stress-related, Becker was more than willing to accept that diagnosis. Why do you think she was so unquestioning? Can you imagine reacting similarly? Becker says denial is a legitimate coping mechanism. Is there truth to her claim?

7. We live in a highly verbal society—talk, talk, talk. How did Becker cope when she lost her ability to speak? Can you imagine such a thing happening to you, even if the loss was temporary? How would you cope? If you had to choose between losing your speech, your hearing, or your sight, which would you choose? Would losing your ability to touch or taste be as devastating?

8. Becker's postsurgical experiences with both her neuropsychologist and her speech therapist were funny, cruel, pathetic, horrifying, real. What do you think was most frustrating to Becker? Her inability to speak, read, and draw? Her inability to get others to understand how frustrated she was? Or the fact that no one could tell her how long her recovery would take? Have you ever been in a similar situation? Were you most scared by not being able to accomplish something or by not knowing when you would be able to?

9. Many (if not most) memoirs are written years after the experience that inspired them. Becker wrote hers in the throes of her recovery. What is gained and lost by writing in real time?

10. Becker's experience affected all her relationships—with her partner, her family, her friends, her neighbors. Do you believe partners or spouses have a responsibility to stay together during a medical crisis? Is there a time when staying together isn't healthy? How far should friends extend themselves to one another during a crisis? What is a good neighbor?

11. Becker's decision to participate in a bike-a-thon two months after brain surgery was a big one. How did completing the ride contribute to her recovery? Do you think it was an important part of the storyline?

12. Memoir writing is inherently personal, but some authors are more discreet than others. Suzy Becker tells us everything from her age and weight to her sexual feelings. Did you appreciate her candor, or were you made uncomfortable by it? Do you think she ever held back to protect the feelings of family or friends? As a reader, do you draw a line between what is okay to know and what is simply too personal? Can you think of memoirs you've read that have "crossed the line"?

13. A reader's life experience often informs his or her reaction to a story. Do you think people who have had brain trauma or surgery and those who haven't will respond to the book in the same way? How does your personal experience affect your reading of autobiography? Other works of nonfiction or fiction? Which do you prefer, a book that mirrors your experience or one that allows you to see into someone else's?